Integrating Arts Therapies into Education

This book offers a variety of effective, concrete ways to better assimilate arts therapies in the educational system.

Featuring leading art therapists and the models they have honed as a result of their arts experience in education, *Integrating Arts Therapies into Education* discusses systemic issues and challenges related to work in the education system such as confidentiality, multidisciplinary teamwork with educators and contact with parents. Divided into two parts, the first discusses systemic issues related to work in the education system, and the second presents a series of dedicated models that can be implemented in the education system. Each chapter consists of a theoretical background, a description of the working model, a clinical example or case study and a summary.

Creative arts and expressive therapy practitioners will find this guide filled with the most effective ways to approach and deliver arts therapies in a school setting.

Dafna Regev is an art therapist and researcher. She is a senior lecturer and member of the Emili Sagol Creative Arts Therapies Research Center at the University of Haifa, Israel.

Sharon Snir is an art therapist and researcher. She is an associate professor and head of the art therapy masters program at Tel Hai College, Israel.

Integrating Arts Therapies into Education

A Collective Volume

Edited by

Dafna Regev and Sharon Snir

Translated by Dalya Weisbrod

Routledge
Taylor & Francis Group
NEW YORK AND LONDON

Originally published in Hebrew as:
"When the Creative Arts Therapies and the Israeli Education System Meet: Features and Applications"

https://www.haifa.ac.il/index.php/he/
http://catrc.haifa.ac.il

First published in English 2021
by Routledge
605 Third Avenue, New York, NY 10158

and by Routledge
2 Park Square, Milton Park, Abingdon, Oxon, OX14 4RN

Routledge is an imprint of the Taylor & Francis Group, an informa business

Original edition published 2018 by University of Haifa: Emili Sagol – Creative Arts Therapies Research Center (Israel)

Library of Congress Cataloging-in-Publication Data
A catalog record for this title has been requested

ISBN: 978-0-367-44208-8 (hbk)
ISBN: 978-0-367-44207-1 (pbk)
ISBN: 978-1-003-00832-3 (ebk)

Typeset in Garamond
by Deanta Global Publishing Services, Chennai, India

Contents

Contributors

Ayalon, Anat Art therapist (M.A.), parent-child therapist and CBT psychotherapist, supervisor and lecturer.

Belity, Irit Art therapist (M.A.), clinical supervisor, and arts therapies coordinator at a special education school. Lecturer and supervisor at the University of Haifa, School of Creative Arts Therapies, and Kibbutzim College. Has a private clinic.

Bruno, Yael Art therapist (M.A.), Jungian sandplay therapist (ISST), and parent-child therapist. Clinical supervisor and coordinator in the Druze town of Isafia. Lecturer in para-medical and art therapies at Oranim College.

Court, Deborah (Ph.D.), Associate Professor, School of Education, Bar-Ilan University.

Dvir, Osnat Art therapist (M.A.) in primary education, specializes in the open-studio approach in primary schools.

Frieman, Nava Drama therapist (M.A.), social worker. Clinical supervisor and regional arts therapies coordinator for the Israel Board of Education and has a private clinic.

Goldman, Sandra Art therapist (M.A.) in the religious Jewish education and pre-school sector.

Halahmi, Yael Art therapist (M.A.) in the public education sector, specializes in co-therapy groups in special education classes.

Heller, Anat Drama therapist (Ph.D.), lecturer and supervisor at the Art and Drama therapies training program at Tel Hai College. One of the founders and a staff member of the open studio at "Ziv" hospital. Owns a private clinic.

Kalfus, Yael Art therapist (M.A.) at the Rehabilitation Educational Medical Day Care Center at Alyn Hospital, and at Maale Erev, a high school for teenage drop-outs in Jerusalem.

Liban, Anat Art therapist (M.A.), couple and family therapist in public education and private clinic, and Chairperson of the Visual Arts Therapy division of YAHAT (The Israel Association for Creative Arts Therapies).

Mann, Tal Music therapist (M.A.) and psychotherapist at the Rehabilitation Educational Medical Day Care Center at Alyn Hospital, and Hosen-Efrat, a national therapeutic center. Has a private clinic.

Massarwa, Zakiah Art therapist (M.A.) at the Educational Center in Schneider Children's Medical Center, Chairperson of the Arab Society Division of YAHAT (The Israel Association for Creative Arts Therapies).

Nissimov-Nahum, Edna Art therapist (Ph.D.), clinical supervisor, lecturer and academic program director, affiliated with the Ministry of Education and The David Yellin Academic College of Education.

Ofer-Yarom, Mickey (Ph.D.). Art therapist, clinical supervisor. Teaching at the Department of Special Education, Faculty of Education, Kibbutzim College, Tel-Aviv.

Raubach Kaspy, Racheli Art therapist (M.A.) at the Counseling and Treatment Division for Youth, Golan Regional Council and the Bait Bakfar Kinneret senior living home.

Regev, Dafna Art therapist (Ph.D.) and researcher. Senior lecturer and member of the Emili Sagol Creative Arts Therapies Research Center at the University of Haifa.

Roginsky, Efrat Music therapist (Ph.D.), clinical supervisor and regional arts therapies coordinator for the Israel Board of Education. Lecturer at the School of Creative Arts Therapies at the University of Haifa.

Sade-Dor, Tamar Art therapist (M.A.) in higher education and special education. Specializing in the open-studio approach in Autism.

Shamir, Adina (Ph.D.) Associate Professor, Head of Ph.D. Committee, Director of the Center for Technology in Special Education, Head of the Special Education program (B.A.), Bar Ilan University.

Snir, Sharon Art therapist (Ph.D.) and researcher. Associate professor and Head of the Art Therapy M.A. Program at Tel Hai College.

Tamir, Rona Dyadic Art therapist and psychotherapist (M.A.) at the "Hosen-resilience" center in Sderot. Supervisor in the educational system and lecturer at the Musrara school of photography and Psagot Therapists' Training Institute.

Ulitzur-Zemel, Michal Art therapist and psychotherapist, supervisor, lecturer and coordinator of the MAAT program and the practicum program at the David Yellin Academic College. Has a private clinic.

Yoel, Haggai Animal-assisted therapist and group instructor (M.A.). Manager of the Eyal Farm, an ecological and therapeutic farm at Kibbutz Ramat Rachel.

Preface

Arts therapy in the education system sounds like a distant dream for arts therapists in many countries. Workshops that we have been organized in international conferences in recent years have exposed us to the concerns of arts therapists who are currently making enormous efforts to gain a foothold in the education system. In Israel, however, the situation is different. Today, more than 3,500 arts therapists work within the education system. This means that there is an arts therapist in almost every school and that they have been mandated officially to provide emotional support for students in need.

Since 2013 we have been conducting studies on the role and efficacy of arts therapies in the education system. This has led to an in-depth grasp of the complexities of integrating a therapeutic profession into the educational sector. The outcome of these studies clearly confirms the potential of working with students in arts therapies within the framework in which they spend so many hours of their day. Yet, much work remains to be done to exploit this potential and overcome these complexities.

During the many encounters we have had with professionals in the field, we saw that despite the obstacles to integrating this therapeutic profession within the educational system, arts therapists have initiated many wonderful projects and found specific solutions to the problems in the field to achieve meaningful work within the education system. However, these solutions have not been disseminated because they are not documented in the literature, and therefore often remain at the local level. Our desire to make these discoveries, models, programs and insights widely available prompted us to write this book. Its overall aim is to contribute to the discourse in the field by sharing the important work done by arts therapists within the educational system. This discourse is relevant to arts therapists who work in the education system as well as teachers who are interested in making a meaningful connection with arts therapists.

The book has two parts. The first deals with the systemic aspects of work in the education system. The chapters describe the complexity of arts therapy in school, its importance, and put forward possible solutions. In the first chapter, the art therapist Anat Ayalon describes a model that she developed to enable arts therapists to work better together with educators. In the second chapter, Irit Belity, an art therapist, focuses on arts therapists' work with parents in the school system. The third chapter was written by drama therapist Nava Frieman and deals with the complexity of maintaining therapeutic confidentiality in the school system. In the fourth chapter, art therapists Michal Ulitzur-Zemel, Yael Kalfus, Tal Mann and animal assistant therapist Haggai Yoel present a model to integrate arts therapies into a multidisciplinary team in a school operating in a long-term care hospital. The fifth and final chapter in this part relates to multiculturalism in the education system. Art therapists Yael Bruno and Zakiah Massarwa describe the encounter between arts therapists and clients from different cultures.

The second part deals with dedicated working models in the education system to cope with the specific characteristics of this system. The sixth chapter by art therapists Dafna Regev and Rona Tamir describes a parent-child art psychotherapy model developed in recent years as part of school arts therapy. In the seventh chapter, drama therapist Anat Heller describes the open studio as a model for individual artwork in a group setting in schools, which she also researched in her Ph.D. dissertation. In the eighth chapter, art therapist Edna Nissimov-Nahum presents a model she developed for working with students who act out aggressively in educational settings. In chapter nine, art therapist Mickey Ofer-Yarom, in collaboration with Deborah Court and Adina Shamir describe a model for group-class arts therapy that was also researched in her Ph.D. dissertation. In the tenth chapter, art therapist Anat Liban describes a model for exhibiting artworks by art therapy clients in the school space. In the eleventh chapter, music therapist Efrat Roginsky, together with art therapists Tamar Sade-Dor, Osnat Dvir, Yael Halahmi and Sandra Goldman describes projects stemming from the conceptualization of the therapeutic practice in school as community-based arts therapies. The twelfth and final chapter is devoted to the role of substitutes where arts therapists are on maternity leave in the education system. Art therapists Sharon Snir and Racheli Raubach Kaspy draw on Raubach Kaspy's M.A. thesis on this topic.

Many examples depicting clients in therapy are presented throughout this book. Most are composites of clients that the authors of each chapter have treated over the years. In cases where a specific client is described, written consent was obtained from both the client and his or her parents. Note that all names are pseudonyms to protect the clients' confidentiality and anonymity.

We hope this book will be of value to arts therapists and educational staff in their collaborative work, be useful to students in arts therapy training taking their first steps in the field and serve as an inspiration for developing more models and continuing to document existing ones more fully and broadly.

Acknowledgments

We would like to thank the many people for their time and efforts in the preparation of this book. First and foremost, we are indebted to all the arts therapists who contributed to the writing of this book. Your wealth of knowledge inspired us to embark on this project. We are grateful to the three Israel Department of Education national arts therapist supervisors (past and present): Tami Yermiyahu, Anat Marnin-Shaham and Anat Mendelson who helped structure the content to this book. We would like to thank the Emili Sagol Creative Arts Therapies Research Center for funding the Hebrew version of this book. We are especially grateful to Prof. Rachel Lev-Wiesel and Danielle Friedlander.

We would like to thank Dalya Weisbrod, an art therapist and proficient translator, for the translation of this book. We would also like to acknowledge the superlative assistance we received from our publisher, Taylor & Francis, and specifically Amanda Devine, who guided us through the whole process.

Finally, this is a wonderful opportunity to thank our dear families: the Regev family, Alon, Maya, Inbal, Adi and Shai, and Dafna's parents Edna and Michael Neuberger, and the Snir family, Yehuda, Michal, Shira and Nami, and Sharon's parents Gila and the late Jehuda Livne. Your support and love throughout continue to give meaning to our work.

Part I

Systemic Aspects of Work in the Education System

1 The Collaborative Arts Therapist-Teacher Model

Theory and Practice

Anat Ayalon

Introduction

The work of an arts therapist in the school setting addresses the constant to and fro between the inner world expressed in the therapy room and the external reality that exists in the school space. Transitioning between the classroom and the therapy room often requires flexibility and the ability to bridge between the therapeutic and educational languages. The collaborative working Arts Therapist-Teacher model presented in this chapter was designed to connect these two spaces and optimize the therapeutic process taking place in the educational system. It incorporates therapeutic work with the student, joint work on the part of the arts therapist and teacher in terms of collaborative thinking and training sessions, as well as joint sessions involving the teacher and the student in the presence of the arts therapist. In this collaborative working model, the student enjoys a personal relationship with the arts therapist and the teacher, thus expanding the therapeutic space beyond the confines of the therapy room and into the school space. The implementation of this collaborative work as a function of this model reinforces arts therapy by empowering both the client (student) and the educational staff.

Theoretical Background

In recent years, increasing numbers of students in the education system are diagnosed with Attention Deficit (Hyperactivity) Disorder (ADD/ADHD), impulsive behavior or Oppositional Defiant Disorder (ODD). Integrating these students into the educational system is not a straightforward process, and they often struggle to control their emotional experiences. Rebellious or aggressive behavior is occasionally a way to avoid confronting overwhelming emotions (Chethik, 2003). Many of these children who are referred to arts therapies within the school framework find it difficult to control and regulate their behavior. The goal of arts therapy is to provide emotional support and help these students improve their academic performance.

In general, the purpose of arts therapy within the education system is to assist and ease students' adjustment process to the educational framework and reduce the emotional barriers that hinder learning. At the turn of the millennium, the World Health Organization (2001) outlined a biopsychosocial model for therapists in the health professions. This model links the medical and environmental components of individuals with special needs and considers the functioning of the individual and the difficulties faced to be the outcome of dynamic interactions between health conditions and environmental, social and cultural factors (Garbarino, 1992; Greenberg et al., 2003). Students' behavior is influenced and shaped by the environment; hence it is impossible to evaluate a student's behavior without observing him or her in a range of environments. Approaches that view the development of the individual as a series of life cycles underscore the importance of interventions in the medical, emotional, social and environmental arenas. They also emphasize the importance of the integration and joint activities of the staff in each of these areas. This perception of the importance of systemic teamwork forms the groundwork for the collaborative working model associating the arts therapist with the educational team proposed in this chapter. Arts therapy within the educational system addresses the emotional and interpersonal aspects of students' functioning. In the educational setting, therapists can observe students outside the therapy room, which can lead to a better understanding of the nature of their interpersonal interactions in different social settings.

The need to address the therapeutic aspects of these different spheres prompted me to search for ways to engage the educational staff in promoting arts therapy for students. Arts therapies in the education system are part of an overall vision of students' optimal integration into school life educationally, socially and emotionally from kindergarten onward.

The arts therapist's work in schools and pre-schools has three key features: (1) The arts therapist engages with clients in a setting where they spend a great deal of time for many years. (2) The arts therapist aims to identify difficulties in students' development and encourage the proactive implementation of solutions. (3) Arts therapists who work in the education system are the fulcrum for three systems: the family, the education system and the student's personality (Osterville, 1995). There is an overwhelming consensus (e.g., Proulx, 2003) that parents are essential to the success of the therapeutic process in children. Therefore, working with parents has become more prevalent in therapeutic work in schools. However, this is often not possible, and the therapeutic intervention is largely implemented with the student separately, without the involvement of the social or family systems. This is due to the lack of sufficient therapy hours, a lack of parental awareness of the need for therapy for their children and even a lack of parental awareness of the availability of therapy in the educational setting. Typically, we meet with parents at most two or three times during the academic year (see Belity, Chapter 2). Is it possible to work with a student without the involvement of his/her parents? Is it possible to achieve significant change with one weekly arts therapy session? The answers to these questions are complex. The reality is that in many cases we are able to accomplish meaningful processes of change, alleviate those feelings that hinder integration and help these students integrate with their peers despite the lack of substantial parental involvement (Case & Dalley, 2002).

When implementing a collaborative working model, the differences between the therapeutic language and the educational language must be taken into consideration. Becoming acquainted and conducting preliminary work sessions are essential to creating an inter-professional dialogue. A collaborative working method supports the therapeutic process significantly but demands a greater level of commitment on the part of the teacher to actively listen to the student and work with the arts therapist, who engages in a dialogue with the teacher to accompany, contain and guide him/her.

The alliance between the teacher and the arts therapist is contracted for the sake of the student and has several notable benefits. First, the student is exposed to a "therapist-teacher" relationship that allows him/her to feel supported by overall systemic attention and interest. The second benefit relates to the ability to maintain continuous therapist-teacher communication. The teacher regularly updates the arts therapist about life events that the students and their families go through, as well as unusual events that occur at school. The teacher interacts with the student for several hours a day and is aware of his/her difficulties and strengths. The events in the students' lives affect their emotions and can lead to different, and at times, unusual behavior. With the help of the teacher, the arts therapist gets to know the student in his/her daily environment and learns about these life events. Updated reports by the teacher as to positive experiences, such as the birth of a sibling or moving, which can cause students to feel uncertain and occasionally have ambiguous feelings, are significant and can help the arts therapist assess the nature of behavioral changes and process these experiences with the student. These updates are important to bridging between the arts therapy room and the outside world. At the same time, the arts therapist, who meets the student individually in the therapy room, is privy to aspects of the student's life that are often not seen outside of therapy, and can also share certain information with the teacher (for more on confidentiality issues, see Chapter 3). This exchange of information enables the teacher to become familiar with the way students experience the world and have a better understanding of what motivates their behavior. The information provided by the arts therapist is conveyed solely for purposes of dialogue and is limited to the needs of the student; personal content that emerges during therapy remains undisclosed to preserve the subjective needs of the student while providing a window on external reality.

The teacher's willingness to commit to the therapeutic model leads to greater collaboration and acknowledgment of the role of the therapeutic process. This acknowledgment is of utmost importance and may help avoid situations common to many schools where the arts therapist does not get good quality support from the education system (Snir et al., 2018). When this type of exchange does not take place, this can hinder the circulation of information between the teacher and the arts therapist. For example, the educational staff may not inform the arts therapist of school activities that conflict with a therapy schedule or may not let the therapist know that the student has had a tough day and needs help organizing and mustering strength for the rest of the day.

Collaborative work with the teacher allows for manifestations of empathy for the students and their problems, but also allows the teachers who interact with them on a daily basis to express their concerns. The teacher's empowerment and accompaniment in sessions with the arts therapist during their collaborative work and their discussions about the teacher's own difficulties in working with the student may enable these teachers to deal better with them because they are given the space to express their difficulties. I believe in the strength of such dialogues and during my work I have discovered that this space in fact provides another containing space for the student in therapy. This may enable the teacher to assist the student in the transition from his or her personal space to the reality of the classroom. The arts therapist's interaction with the teacher can develop into another safe space for the student beyond the therapy room.

In arts therapy sessions, students confront emotional difficulties. These issues are acknowledged, and a space is created to deal with them and learn ways of coping with them, as well as a variety of possible alternative behaviors (Nissimov-Nahum, 2008). In the working model, the teacher and the arts therapist are only exposed to some of the students' emotional content and behaviors in different contexts, and both also understand the importance of systemic work that completes the picture.

Description of the Working Model

The model presented in this chapter combines arts therapist-teacher work in parallel with therapeutic work. Its aim is to maximize the effectiveness of the therapeutic process for students within the school setting, and to develop an awareness of their feelings and behaviors by bridging between the therapeutic and classroom experiences. The novelty of this model lies in its routine integration of collaborative work between the arts therapist and the teacher, and the impact of these exchanges on individual arts therapy sessions between the therapist and the student.

In the first stage, before the therapeutic process commences, I hold an intake session with the student's parents. The purpose of this session is to obtain information about the student's medical, emotional and developmental condition, as well as information about their integration in family life and in their social surroundings. During the intake session, the parents sign a consent form allowing their child to receive arts therapy in the school setting.

Soon afterwards, the first session with the teacher takes place. In this session, I outline my rationale for the importance of our collaborative work and emphasize its significance to the therapeutic process. Throughout this discussion, the importance of the teacher's role is highlighted as the student's main accompanying figure during the week who can be a fulcrum for change in the student's behavior. Acknowledgment of the importance of the teacher's role and understanding the implications of the teacher's engagement in the process and contribution to the fulfillment of the therapeutic goals are ways of confirming the teacher's commitment to the process. During this first meeting, we agree to a contract which outlines our collaborative working model. This includes setting a regular time slot for future meetings and deciding on the nature of our exchanges about the student. Special emphasis is placed on the importance of maintaining confidentiality.

Ensuring the teacher's awareness of the issue of student privacy is crucial. Teachers often share complex stories and experiences in the staffroom about specific students who exhibit challenging behaviors. The teachers' need to share and unload their daily interactions and experiences is an obvious one, since most of the time they have to deal with classroom behavior on their own. However, with respect to students who are in therapy, the collaborative model provides teachers an opportunity to use these meetings as a place to speak out about experiences and difficulties which also prompts them to avoid talking about the students in public spaces such as the school corridors. The first meeting also explores initial ideas that can lead to a common goal, starting from becoming aware of the student and showing empathy until a therapy plan can be formulated.

During the first therapy session with the student, I assess his/her difficulties in different frameworks, including the school setting. I define a contract which emphasizes the rules of conduct in the arts therapy room, including issues such as mutual respect, using the art equipment properly and a pledge to maintain confidentiality. Upholding the confidentiality of therapy is one of the pillars of the professional code of ethics that arts therapists must adhere to and is essential to maintaining trust between the student and the therapist. However, working within the educational system places the arts therapist in a position where he/she also needs to share information with the multidisciplinary staff who referred the student to therapy. I ask all students in therapy how they would feel about my talking to their teachers. I discuss what is shared and with whom in terms of the content that emerges during the sessions. I emphasize that the arts therapy room is a safe place for them and that the content and behavior that emerges during therapy will remain in the therapy room and between us. I also note that working with the teacher enables further support for the therapeutic process and the student's optimal integration into the classroom and the educational setting. Students are informed that they will meet individually with the teacher and may also use these sessions to strengthen the educational experience. In addition, we agree on behavior and reactions in times of crisis. For example, if students feel they want to leave the classroom, they need to say so and try to find an acceptable solution with the teacher or the therapist (a number of alternatives are suggested such as comfort blankets, taking a few minutes to calm down in the bathroom or returning to class). I inform the students that I will meet with their teachers and inquire whether there is anything that they would like me to ask or if they would like me to convey a message from them.

In the conversations when both the teacher and the student are present, the basis for behavior change is also examined and the client's experience as a student in the classroom and as part of a peer group are discussed in detail. Student and teacher also enter into a contract that ensures that all content will remain confidential. This type of conversation helps the teacher observe all the qualities of the student and not just classroom behavior, and thus creates a more secure space between the two.

The meetings with the teacher are held once every two weeks in conjunction with the therapeutic work. These exchanges help create a consistent language for use when responding to the student, and also ensure that the therapeutic and the educational efforts are in sync. The goal is to help the teacher adjust and formulate different responses to different students. Our work sessions are in fact comparable to training sessions: I try to explain the reasons for specific behavior and reflect the students' feelings, which are at times hidden behind their mode of conduct (for example, aggressive or confrontational behavior). In addition, I guide the teacher and recommend specific responses to the students' behavior. For example, if students start fidgeting, the teacher can approach them, touch their shoulders and look into their eyes. If the student misbehaves, the teacher can respond: "I can see that you're angry, but you can't kick the chair."

In the sessions with the teacher, the exchange of information focuses on the core elements of the student's particular issues, as well as coping methods and insights gained from the arts therapy room. The arts therapist avoids emphasizing direct content that exposes the therapeutic process that could potentially undermine progress and is not necessarily required to clarify the central themes. The arts therapist's objective is to consult, resolve and make decisions, and clarify methods of intervention to understand the student and the progression of the related educational/therapeutic goals. For example, in cases of bullying or social ostracism, family difficulties or manifestations of emotional distress, the message to the teacher is that the student currently requires more empathy than usual and is experiencing difficulty.

This multipronged work evolves out of the outward-oriented learning process and the inward-oriented arts therapy process (Case & Dalley, 2002). In my experience, cases in which the students' learning ability is compromised due to internal conflicts requires work that merges individual therapeutic sessions along with building a positive student-teacher relationship to achieve a successful outcome. The model enables systemic work and expands the therapeutic space to occupy more hours while jointly considering the needs of the student and communicating with the school staff in order to maximize these clients' functioning as students and as social beings.

This model can be enacted in individual therapy sessions with the student's teacher or in a group session with the entire team that works with these students in the school. It is also possible to develop and present the therapeutic work to the multidisciplinary school staff in cases where one student's reason for referral to arts therapy also manifests in similar behavior in other students.

Clinical Example

Danny (collective pseudonym that does not refer to one specific student) was referred to art therapy for rebellious behavior accompanied by outbursts of rage and physical and verbal violence. He was not interested in learning and was an underachiever. In the classroom he did not participate. Danny came to class without the right books or material and did not do his homework. He wiggled a lot in his seat, played with objects, and would move around and take papers from his peers in class. When other students reacted, he would reply indignantly: "What do you want? I hardly took anything!" and when the teacher would comment, he would react angrily: "You always pick on me!" Occasionally he even kicked his chair and left the classroom, slamming the door behind him. During recess, Danny played football with his classmates as a midfielder. He would run from side to side while barking instructions to the other players. The game was often accompanied by friction with the other players, where Danny would get angry and complain about the players' performance, but others expressed complaints about Danny physically pushing the other players.

During her two years with the class, the teacher had tried numerous ways of reducing the intensity of Danny's behavior. She tried to encourage him or alternatively punish him, engaged in different kinds of contracts with him and his parents, but none had an effect that lasted more than a few days.

The decision to treat Danny according to the "Arts therapist-Teacher" working model was suggested after many attempts at therapy that had failed to produce satisfactory behavioral change. Although the therapeutic process took place in the art therapy room, the teacher also met with Danny in individual sessions where she addressed his behavioral tendencies and was empathetic to his difficulties. Later, they discussed what could help him in times of crisis, and even agreed on a secret signal that allowed Danny to leave the classroom for a few minutes without interrupting the lesson.

During the arts therapist-teacher work sessions, we addressed several points: (1) We assessed events that took place in the classroom and in the yard at recess. (2) Recommendations were suggested for ways of responding to Danny's behavior in the classroom, and time was spent thinking about the nature of the teacher's individual sessions with Danny. (3) The teacher was given a space to express her emotions about her work with Danny. After a year of collaborative work with the teacher, I realized that we had progressed towards achieving our therapeutic goals in a shorter time period than in similar cases without using the model.

During the first session with his teacher, Danny was skeptical. He barely spoke and he apparently felt that he was being reprimanded. However, the continuity of their sessions and their discussions gradually led to a level of intimacy and trust. Danny managed to wait until his next private session with the teacher before expressing any social or educational issues that transpired during the week. Simultaneously, during the art therapy sessions, Danny was given a space to express his concerns, his lack of trust and his difficult feelings.

The interaction between the student and the teacher was respectful and considerate on both sides, and more so than the year before. In my view, this testifies to the change in the teacher's attitude and the set responses to the student by the entire educational staff in the past. These contributed significantly to the decrease in Danny's disruptive behavior. He apparently felt calmer, managed to compose himself better, had more positive learning experiences, managed to stay in the classroom during lessons and improved in his academic performance and social functioning. As part of this effort, steps were taken to integrate Danny within the school system, and to encourage the individuation of his inner experiences. The collaborative work created an alliance between colleagues who had shared responsibility for the process. The teacher's sensitivity and commitment to the process should not be taken for granted. I was excited that we were able to create a training framework, as well as continuous exchanges throughout the year, and felt the mutual commitment we both shared to achieve behavioral change.

Summary and Conclusions

Arts therapy with kindergarten and elementary school children takes place primarily in educational frameworks. The therapeutic process in the educational system needs to consider the different systems that influence the child's development: the family system, the educational system, as well as the characteristics of the child's personality. Throughout my work in the school setting as an art therapist, I have come to realize that the combination of arts therapy work and the work of other professionals in school facilitates creating a non-judgmental capacity to observe students behind their "disruptive behavior." The discussions and frequent meetings with the classroom teachers of students I treated enabled the progression of systemic work and extended the therapeutic space to incorporate more hours and more spaces in which the student spends time. During our meetings, the teacher and I thought jointly about the needs of the students and there was communication with the school staff to maximize their functioning as students and as social beings.

Arts therapy in the education system should integrate aspects of individual therapy at the systemic level. The difficulty of merging the two systems stems from the fundamental differences in the perception of the causes of the issues at hand, the nature of the changes in the student and the type of therapy. In individual therapy, the source of student's difficulties is viewed as originating from within the individual (and is described as conflict, impairment, illness and so on), whereas in therapy at a systemic level, the root cause of the difficulty is perceived as the result of interactions created by individuals and the structure of their relationships.

My experience also shows me that this model has several difficulties and limitations that deserve mention:

1. Ethics and confidentiality within and outside the arts therapy room. There is a conflict concerning the extent to which the teacher participates in the therapeutic process and the way in which the collaborative work should be implemented. Therapists need to be aware of the importance of continuously maintaining client privacy, in particular when working with teachers in the collaborative working model.
2. Professional exposure of the arts therapist. The arts therapist emerges from the protected and private therapy room and agrees to conduct an open discussion, share therapeutic concerns and notions, and the intervention techniques employed. This exposure may also prompt criticism or hesitation from the teacher and the educational staff regarding the nature of the arts therapy process.
3. The possibility of competition for prestige between the arts therapist and the teacher. This type of rivalry can center around the issue of which of the two professionals knows the student best or who generated the significant changes. Often, the argument is made that in individual or group therapy settings, it is easier to deal with problematic behaviors and achieve change as compared to the teacher who is dealing with 30 or more children in the classroom. Therapeutic tools and professional therapeutic insights are provided by the arts therapist, but a professional and non-egocentric conversation to concretize the aim of working together will reduce the eventuality of power struggles in this setting.
4. Deciding upon a weekly hourly meeting between the arts therapist and the teacher. A joint meeting should take place at a suitable time for both parties while taking into account that the scheduling of this hourly meeting is not straightforward.

Despite these limitations, the benefits I have found and described above lend weight to the value of this working model and the results that it has achieved. The outcomes have had an influence on my own professional development and dignity, as well as the teachers with whom I work.

References

Case, C., & Dalley, T. (Eds.). (2002). *Working with children in art therapy*. London: Routledge.

Chethik, M. (2003). *Techniques of child therapy: Psychodynamic strategies*. New York: Guilford Press.

Garbarino, J. (1992). *Children and families in the social environment*. New York: Routledge.

Greenberg, M.T., Weissberg, R.P., O'Brien, M.U., Zins, J.E., Fredericks, L., Resnik, H., & Elias, M.J. (2003). Enhancing school-based prevention and youth development through coordinated social, emotional, and academic learning. *American Psychologist*, *58*(6–7), 466.

Nissimov-Nahum, E. (2008). A model for art therapy in educational settings with children who behave aggressively. *The Arts in Psychotherapy*, *35*(5), 341–348

Osterville, Z. (1995). *Open solutions: Psychological therapy of the child and his environment*. Jerusalem: Schocken Publishing. (in Hebrew).

Proulx, L. (2003). *Strengthening emotional ties through parent-child-dyad art therapy: Interventions with infants and preschoolers*. London: Jessica Kingsley Publishers.

Snir, S., Regev, D., Keinan, V., Abd El Kader-Shahada, H., Salamey, A., Mekel, D., ... Alkara, M. (2018). Art therapy in the Israeli education system–a qualitative meta-analysis. *International Journal of Art Therapy*, *23*(4), 169–179.

World Health Organization – The World health report: 2001: Mental health : new understanding, new hope. https://www.who.int/whr/2001/en/

2 Working with Parents within the Education System

Irit Belity

Introduction

Many approaches to treating children consider parental involvement to be crucial to the therapeutic process and link the effectiveness of therapy to the parents' extent of cooperation in this process. This chapter describes the therapist-parent relationship[1] in the specific setting of the educational system. It reviews arts therapists' perceptions of the relationship with their clients' parents and the parents' perceptions of this relationship, and then provides examples illustrating arts therapist-parent sessions at key milestones during the academic year. Dedicated working models and ways to implement them in the education system are presented.

Theoretical Background

Arts Therapists' Perceptions of Their Relationship with Clients' Parents

Winnicott stated that "there is no such thing as an infant" (Winnicott, 1965, p. 39), implying that without maternal care, there would be no infant. Winnicott was one of the first theorists to promote parental involvement in children's therapeutic processes. He argued that psychoanalytic research also supports collaboration with parents and the family especially at the two important developmental crossroads of early childhood and adolescence (Winnicott, 1965). Research in developmental psychology has confirmed that children's mental health is affected by their relationship with their parents, their parents' attitudes, beliefs and conduct, and the home environment. Studies on early intervention programs for high-risk parents suggest that parental child care provided by parents can be improved, but that feasibility remains complex (Cohen, 2006). A wide spectrum of approaches to treating children view parental involvement as paramount to the therapeutic process (Chethik, 2003; Espasa, 2004; Frick, Barry, & Bodin, 2000) and consider that the effectiveness of child therapy may hinge on their parents' involvement (Frick et al., 2000; Regev & Snir, 2014).

Today, the prevailing professional approach in the arts therapies is to involve parents in the therapeutic process. However, for arts therapists working in the educational system, this ideal may be hard to achieve. Some of the hurdles are related to conditions in the educational framework, but other factors are related to the multiple responsibilities of the arts therapist. Arts therapists need to grapple with heavy caseloads, the insufficient number of hours allocated for sessions with clients' parents, the obligation to write up reports, as well as the need to attend professional and multidisciplinary meetings and receive supervision (Belity, Regev & Snir, 2017; Snir et al., 2018). Arts therapists' own seniority and experience, professional identity, personality, therapeutic approach and perception of the parents' role also affect their relationship with their clients' parents. Supervisors who interact with novice and senior arts therapists have noted that seniority status and therapeutic experience influence the extent of contact with clients' parents. Less experienced arts therapists, who have not yet established their professional identity, occasionally feel less comfortable talking to parents (Regev & Snir, 2014; Shamri-Zeevi, Regev, & Snir, 2015). Some are inexperienced in talking with parents, and others feel that since they are not yet mothers/fathers themselves, they do not have the experience to provide guidance to parents. This in turn affects their attitudes and perseverance in encouraging parents to attend meetings or dealing with those who avoid parental guidance sessions (Belity et al., 2017; Nissimov-Nahum, 2008).

Another factor is the arts therapist's therapeutic approach. Some arts therapists consider that therapy should only be carried out in the therapy room irrespective of the client's school and/or home environment. This implies that the therapist relates exclusively to the process unfolding in therapy with the student without consultation or sessions with the educational staff or parents. The content of parental sessions is another issue. Some arts therapists expect to acquire information from the client's parents, but do not reciprocate by sharing their knowledge and insights about the student and his/her functioning, and/or do not provide the parents with practical advice on how to deal with their child. This stance can affect the parents' willingness to attend follow-up meetings. The arts therapist's perceptions of the parents also affect their willingness to initiate meetings. Situations in which the arts therapist is perceived as angry, disappointed, critical or judgmental of the parents may make it difficult for him/her to encourage them to attend meetings and to express empathy and appreciation for their efforts.

Parents' Perceptions of Their Relationship with Arts Therapists in the Education System

Alongside the attitudes and perceptions of arts therapists and the framework in which they work, parents' attitudes are also crucial. Research has shown that parental behavior, in their role as the child's first educators, largely determines the child's drive for achievement, internal locus of control and level of curiosity (Bray, 2001; Wallace, 2013). Parents influence their children's self-image and attitude towards learning and school (Shumow & Miller, 2001). Parents are the most significant figures in the child's life, and it has been recommended to develop a stronger relationship between parents and the educational setting for the benefit of the child (Lee & Bowen, 2006). Research suggests that the more parents engage in their children's education, the more likely their children will do well in school (Harris & Goodall, 2008). Parental involvement has been positively associated with student grade point averages (Gutman & Midgley, 2000).

The relationship between the parents, the educational system and the arts therapists who work in it depends to a great extent on the perception of both sides as to the nature, quality and importance of their relationship (Nissimov-Nahum, 2008). The ideal situation is when parents view the educational-therapeutic staff as partners and allies and as a significant resource for their children. In this case the staff is also likely to perceive the parents as supportive of the child and the entire system. Problems arise when parents are dissatisfied and perceive the staff as service providers they can criticize or attack. Alternatively, parents may view the educational-therapeutic staff as rivals in the education of their children. At other times, parents report that the educational staff takes a critical or judgmental approach and feel that they are being pressured to accept solutions for their children they may not fully endorse, such as prescription medication.

Parents who do not identify with the goals of the education system refrain from close contact with teachers and arts therapists and convey a problematic message to their children (Green et al., 2007). Friedman's (2011) Identification-Awareness theory posits that the level of parental involvement in education is determined by the integration of the level of parental identification with the educational goals, combined with the level of parental awareness of what is taking place in the system. Friedman suggested that parents relate to the school in five different ways: alienation, avoidance, moderate involvement, over-involvement and involvement without identification. He claimed that the optimal level should be moderate involvement combined with identification with the system and a sensitivity to its requirements as well as their child's needs.

It remains unclear what drives parental attitudes towards an educational framework. From my experience in the field, some of the prime motivating factors are the parents' level of awareness of their children's feelings and difficulties, their boundaries with their children and their own self-awareness. These factors dictate the nature of the encounter between parents and the educational staff. Cohen (2006) defined the level of parental awareness as a set of considerations that underlie parental decisions and behavior, the way parents think about their child and the way they understand/interpret their child's behavior. Thus, parental awareness is a qualitative measure related to the level of complexity of parental thinking about their child's understanding and the parents' perceptions of their own roles. This includes the parents' reflective capability (mentalization), i.e., a grasp of the inner processes of the mind (Fonagy, Gergely, Jurist, & Target, 2002). For example, egocentric parents with narcissistic personalities, who view their child as an extension of themselves, interpret any criticism of the child as an assault on them, and may respond aggressively when their child is referred for therapy in school. Conformist parents, who expect their child to "be like everyone else," may experience the referral of their child to therapy as singling out or labeling the child and ostracism. Parents who are oversensitive to their children's needs and empathize with their difficulties may be less connected to the needs of the system and tend to overprotect their children. They may develop expectations that the arts therapist will uphold them in their "battle" against the teaching staff (Cohen, 2006).

Another factor affecting parents' attitudes is their own "ghosts" from the past (Fraiberg, 1980). Parents recall their own childhood school experiences, both good and bad, and these can form the basis for their relationship with the educational-therapeutic staff in their children's schools. Parents' anxiety about these encounters may cause them to place the responsibility for their children's educational and behavioral problems on the system, be flooded with recollections of their own learning difficulties or develop a sense of guilt if they feel that their children's problems are in some way genetic (impulsivity, Attention Deficit Disorder, Learning Disabilities, low capability, etc.). They fear an emotional confrontation with their child's difficulties and prefer to deny or repress the problems to avoid confrontation with teachers or arts therapists (Green et al., 2007). Certain parents may be concerned about the disclosure of information (Ishay-Karin, 2004), its dissemination and misuse.

Cultural disparities can also impede the parent-staff relationship. Parents whose cultural backgrounds differ from those of the teacher may feel misunderstood and that they are being patronized and can refuse to cooperate. Immigrant parents may feel that the system does not understand them and does not make sufficient efforts to help them (Green et al., 2007). This is also the case for parents who find it difficult to attend meetings with the therapist during school hours, for financial reasons related to missed hours at work. A study based on interviews with therapeutic and educational professionals showed that cases characterized by multiple difficulties stemming from low socioeconomic background, violence or disintegration of the family structure may be associated with a very low level of parental commitment to therapy, thus making the relationship with parents even more complex (Snir et al., 2018).

Thus overall, both parents and art therapists are cognizant of the hurdles to establishing a relationship within the educational system. Despite this complexity, fruitful encounters do take place and productive relationships benefitting the child in therapy can develop.

Description of the Working Model and Clinical Examples

Regular Meetings throughout the School Year

In recent years, a model that promotes interactions between arts therapists and parents within the school system has been implemented in Israel. Based on my experience in the field and discussions with many supervisors and arts therapists, we have instituted and in certain cases defined an agreement to convene three meetings with parents during the school year: at the beginning (intake), middle and end of the school year. Each meeting has a different goal, as described below in detail.

Intake session. The goal of these meetings is to collect extensive information about the student on current and pervasive difficulties, the student's strengths, development from childhood to the present, the student's functioning in various domains (educational, social, behavioral, emotional), family information, family structure, the parents' perceptions of their child's difficulties and expectations from therapy (Nissimov-Nahum, 2008). At times, new information emerges during this meeting that was previously unknown to the educational staff, as shown in the following example[2]:

> The parents of Dan (pseudonym), a teenager starting art therapy, were invited to an introductory meeting with me. In the end only the mother[3] attended and she seemed distant, hesitant and restrained in her disclosure of information. I had a feeling that she was struggling to keep a secret. Carefully, but also directly, I asked her a few questions and finally the "secret" was revealed: Dan wets his bed at night. He was ashamed and tried to hide it by avoiding sleeping anywhere except at home. This family secret was never discussed but prompted family members to engage in secretive behavior. The mother revealed this secret with mixed feelings: she regretted exposing her son, and repeatedly asked the therapist not to tell the school staff. At the same time, she also seemed a little relieved.

As suggested through this example, this meeting is designed to establish a therapeutic alliance with the parents based on trust, openness and confidence in the arts therapist and in therapy, to encourage parents to support therapy by recognizing its benefits for their children and to create a channel of communication and reciprocity. Individual arts therapists have their own approaches: some exchange phone numbers with parents, and ask them to contact them directly, whereas others prefer to liaise via the teachers. As in the example above, at times there is a split in the information provided to the arts therapist and to the educational staff. The arts therapist may feel conflicted in terms of loyalty to the client and to the school staff but can take the role of mediator. In the intake interview, after the therapist learns more about the larger picture, the parents and the arts therapist try to come to an agreement on the therapeutic goals. This step is essential because the referral of a student for therapy is most often carried out by the educational staff; i.e., the teacher in collaboration with an extended multidisciplinary team. Situations often arise in which parents ask why their child needs therapy. Occasionally, parents struggle to acknowledge or recognize their children's difficulties, since it touches on their own narcissistic difficulties (Espasa, 2004). The therapeutic contract also includes an agreement on the treatment setting: When will the arts therapist meet with the children? Which lesson will the student skip to go to therapy? Will he/she be given individual or group therapy? How often will the arts therapist and the parents meet and for what purpose?

Thus overall, the initial meeting serves to establish trust in the arts therapist and in therapy, to counsel parents, to demonstrate the kind of communication that can take place between parents and the therapist, and to illustrate the benefits of future parental encounters with the therapist. For example:

> Dan's mother, after revealing her son's bed wetting issue and their feelings about it, asked what could be done. She seemed lost, trapped in the secret that had prevented her from seeing how her son could be helped. After asking what steps had been taken in the past, I suggested she go with Dan for a medical check-up and briefly explained the different approaches to enuresis. The mother then seemed more hopeful, compared to her expressions of powerlessness and guilt at the start of the meeting. I also suggested that she should confide in Dan's teacher to find solutions for extra-curricular activities that require sleepovers. Later in the year, we met several more times, and she told me about the steps she had taken and the progress that had been made. Dan's bed wetting had not stopped by the end of the year, but it was no longer something to hide. The mother's efforts had improved her relationship with her son and enabled more open communication in the family and with the educational staff.

Parents frequently raise other questions during the intake sessions. These can include the nature of the content of these meetings, such as what can be asked and the extent to which personal issues are discussed. This is because some of these questions may seem too intrusive to certain parents, particularly when the arts therapists are at the start of their professional careers. In addition, treatment within the educational setting can lead to confusion for both the arts therapists and the parents as to the legitimacy of asking personal questions or sharing personal information. In my experience, it is important to ask substantive questions and to clarify, both broadly and deeply, all issues related to the child that also shed light on the parents' attitudes, steps taken in the past, the parents' perceptions of their child and the extent of the problem. Therapists should be sensitive to the way questions are formulated, as well as the gradual nature of more in-depth probing of a delicate topic. Other questions have to do with the nature of the parent-therapist relationship: How often should parents meet with the therapist? How can the parties involved maintain contact despite the difficulties of making time for meetings, given the therapists' large number of clients and the limited number of work hours allocated to these meetings? Would the parents be willing to come to school more often? Should the therapist insist on having both parents in attendance during these meetings? Should the arts therapist consider direct telephone contact with the parents or only communicate with them indirectly through the teacher? What can be done if the parents call the arts therapist frequently? Will parents cooperate with the therapy? What is the most reasonable way to work with parents in light of the extent of cooperation with the arts therapist?

Other issues relate specifically to the arts therapist. Does he/she have enough background to work with parents? Does he/she have experience working with parents? Can he/she come up with creative solutions when parents cannot attend planned sessions? Is he/she willing to pursue them? How often should these meetings be rescheduled when parents fail to materialize? There is no single answer to these questions, and individual arts therapists need to develop their own work habits consistent with the framework in which they work, their experience and their personal preferences.

The parental intake session is only one part of the information gathering process at the beginning of therapy. There are also intake sessions with the student and meetings with the educational-therapeutic staff (teachers, counselor, psychologist and information from the student's personal file). When the information is fully collated, the therapy begins. Approximately two to four months later, the parents are invited back to school for the mid-year meeting. These meetings are scheduled as a function of the academic calendar to correspond to times when students get their report cards and when academic award ceremonies take place.

Mid-year meeting. This meeting is typically initiated by the arts therapists. The purpose is to provide a general update that does not compromise the client's right to privacy and to get an update about the client's daily life in the family. For example:

> In the middle of the year, about four months after the start of the year, I met with the mother of Mor, a teenager who was in her second year of individual therapy. The girl's father had never attended these meetings and the relationship thus far had been exclusively with the mother. Mor was very quiet in class and at school, avoided classroom and extra-curricular activities, and secluded herself during breaks whereas at home she behaved differently. During the intake session, the mother told me about her tantrums and wild behavior at home that was manifested in protracted bouts of shouting and verbal and physical violence.

I inquired if there had been a change at home and she told me that a significant change had taken place: she and her husband had separated a few weeks earlier. The mother talked about how hard the divorce proceedings were for her and her problems dealing with her troubled daughter. She later added that Mor had a complex relationship with her father, the first time this topic had ever been brought up. Mor's mother and I both felt pain and sadness and a deeper understanding of Mor's emotional world. We ended the conversation with an overview of support options available to Mor's mother and a referral to family therapy, where she could work with her children on the parents' separation, get support, and learn strategies to support them. The mother expressed concerns that she did not want to reveal the "family secret" to anyone else and asked to meet with me a few more times for support. We met once every two weeks for several sessions. When the mother realized she needed parental guidance, she agreed to my recommendation to seek out family therapy.

In the mid-year meetings with the parents, the following questions arise even more frequently: What should be disclosed to the parents about the therapy and the emotional content that emerges? How much information should be revealed? Should the client be aware that this meeting is taking place? Should the client be asked what he/she would like to be said? Again, there are no clear answers to these questions because the situation is complex and depends on many factors. Arts therapists adhere to a code of ethics which stipulates which high-risk situations require disclosure to parents and/or reporting to the authorities. Apart from these cases, the answers to these questions are determined by the arts therapist's role, the therapeutic approach, the framework in which he/she works, the relationship that has been established with the parents, the parents' willingness to share information and the relationship with the client. In most cases, the discussion emerges from the content the parents bring up in the meeting. If the parents or arts therapist wish to discuss content that emerged in therapy, the topic should first be identified and then discussed in general. It is important to note that this issue is fundamentally different for populations of young clients, in kindergarten or elementary school, as compared to adolescents in junior high and high school. Among the latter, confidentiality and privacy are more intrinsic, given the natural processes of adolescent development. For example, adolescent clients should be informed about meetings with their parents, as shown below:

In the mid-year meeting with the parents of a teenage girl, two distressing issues came to the fore: suspicion of irregular eating habits, and provocative dress and behavior as a way to connect with others, alongside an abundance of age-appropriate preoccupations with her external appearance. These issues emerged during encounters with

> the educational staff and in therapy. After much collaborative thinking with the multidisciplinary staff, it was decided that I would try to clarify the situation in a personal conversation with the parents to gauge their level of awareness and perceptions. The parents were slightly suspicious and reacted defensively while feigning cooperation. Nevertheless, it was clear they did not trust me or the educational staff enough. I deliberated about how to raise these emotionally loaded issues. I started by talking about her daily schedule and eating habits. Her parents claimed that her lack of appetite during school hours was due to the effects of her medication. I learned that both parents were aware of her provocative behavior but could not agree on a response. The mother avoided direct action, and the father responded with aggression, firmness and inappropriate punishment. I realized that parental guidance was needed that included discussing more balanced responses to each parent's concerns.

As seen in this example, mid-year meetings provide an opportunity to raise issues that emerge not only during therapy but also in the school setting. In the example, given the parents' suspicion and our intermittent interactions, I avoided trying to understand why the client was acting out in this particular way. This vignette illustrates the difference between therapy in a school setting and therapy in a clinical setting where parents can be convened more frequently, establish trust and gradually open up and process sensitive issues.

Therapy termination meeting. The therapy termination session typically takes place towards the end of the academic year. The purpose is to review the therapeutic process and the changes that the client has experienced, as well as give parents the opportunity to consider the next phase, possible summer frameworks (for at-risk children), and to make recommendations for continued therapy if needed. It is also important to clarify the parents' perceptions of the process their child experienced in therapy, changes in the family and the client's functioning at home, and their thoughts about the future, as shown below:

> Yael is an adolescent with learning disabilities and has a complex family situation. She is currently transitioning between junior high and high school. During the last month of school, she seemed depressed and self-absorbed. In the summary session concluding therapy with her mother, I described her condition, as perceived by the educational-therapeutic staff, and I inquired whether her condition had deteriorated at home as it appeared to have done at school. The mother experienced her daughter differently, and described her as being full of life, happy and socially active. Together we tried to understand why there was such a difference between her behavior at school and at home. One of the possible explanations was her upcoming transition to high school

> and concerns about the academic effort it would require. Yael was also saying goodbye to significant people in her school life: a teacher whom she was close to, some of her friends who were enrolled in other educational frameworks, and also from myself, after three years of working together. It is possible that all these changes weighed heavily on Yael. I restated the importance of continuing with art therapy, which would support Yael's transition to high school. In addition, I met with Yael several times, during which we processed our therapy termination and her transition, along with the complexity of emotions that emerged. I also encouraged her teacher to have a personal conversation with her, and to deal with the separation processes from her class together with all the classmates by devoting time to activities on this theme.

This example illustrates the importance of the relationship between the arts therapist and the parents in acquiring a fuller picture of the client. The conversation with Yael's mother resulted in recommendations concerning Yael and her family, Yael's emotional needs, and systemic recommendations that helped Yael and others in her class experience a smoother and more gradual transition.

Models of the Arts Therapist-parent Relationship under Specific Situations in the Ministry of Education

Three main working models have been formulated in the last decade by the Israeli education system to deal with specific situations when working with parents. The first model, developed by Manor Binyamini (2014), focuses on the transitions children make in the education system: starting school, moving from grade to grade and to different school frameworks (elementary school, middle school, high school). The second model relates to working with parents during times of crisis, and the third model centers on parent-child group therapy that take place in schools or treatment centers.

Manor Binyamini's model (2014) promotes a multidisciplinary teamwork approach specifically for parents of students in special education. This model illustrates the importance of parental sharing in terms of their child's developmental process that acknowledges their intimate knowledge and understanding of their child. In this model, the meetings focus on the three transitions above. The multidisciplinary meetings include staff such as the teacher, counselor, supervisor, arts therapist, psychologist and the parents. The model is broad and refers to the setting in which the meeting takes place, the spoken language (professional jargon and the necessary explanations) and the structure of the meeting (beginning, middle and concluding statements). This model has been successfully implemented in several schools in conjunction with in-person encounters between the arts therapist and parents. The two axes of the meetings are conducted simultaneously: one involves the multidisciplinary team meetings with the parents, and the other is the meeting between the parents and the arts therapist. Together, they form a container for the relationship between the educational and therapeutic staff, and a holding space for the parents and the child. The arts therapist's contribution to these multidisciplinary meetings involves sharing information, engaging in educational-therapeutic processes, conceptualizing emotional issues, and defining and explaining important phenomena, situations and difficulties to the staff and parents.

For example, in the transition to junior high school for a student with special needs, a joint meeting is scheduled between the staff and parents at the beginning of seventh grade in which the parents describe the child, his/her strengths and difficulties. In addition, initial thoughts are shared as how to best help the child. If difficulties arise which should be addressed outside school, the parents are referred to the appropriate frameworks and professionals. Follow-up calls are scheduled as needed. This lets parents get to know the educational-therapeutic team and establish a relationship of trust and cooperation based on reciprocity and shared expectations. At the beginning of the meeting, the student is present. Then, the student is asked to leave the room and the discussion continues with the parents. Below is an example:

> The parents of a student who started seventh grade in a special education class attended an introductory conversation roughly a month after the start of the academic year. The parents were informed that it was a multidisciplinary team meeting. Their son was waiting for them and greeted them indifferently. During the conversation, the student was asked how he felt about his transition to the school. He eagerly described his experience in breathless detail, his relief compared to the previous schools he had attended, and his hopes of making new friends. His parents reacted very differently. While listening, his father recoiled and seemed uncomfortable with what his son was saying, but his mother smilingly encouraged him and seemed glad to hear him express himself. We reflected on the student's description and formed initial mutual expectations with him, by focusing on social goals, as he had suggested. When the student left the room, his father shared his feelings, his difficulties accepting his son, and his struggle to deal with his condition. The mother expressed joy and satisfaction in the way her son depicted himself as aware of his difficulties as well as his academic strengths, and his confidence when he spoke. She was optimistic about his integration into the classroom and school. They both shared their daily problems in dealing with their son and disclosed that they had been receiving parental guidance for many years.

During this one meeting, the drama in the child's relationships with each of his parents was revealed and the beginning of an educational-therapeutic program was initiated. The parents discussed their son's development, previous treatments, family relationships, social relationships and even the parents' family histories. Since the nature of each parent's relationship with the child was openly discussed during the conversation, it enabled the arts therapist to relate to and broaden the content that emerged and discuss it further.

The second model is applied by arts therapists during a crisis situation experienced by a client and his/her parents, and serves as a short-term response. The implementation of the model is influenced by the personality and commitment of the arts therapist, and the framework of therapy. While in most treatments the sessions between the arts therapist and the parents are held approximately three times a year, in this model the meetings can take place on a weekly basis. These sessions take place during the arts therapist's working hours and can continue for several months, as illustrated in the following example.

> Meital, a teenage girl with Autism Spectrum Disorder (ASD), who was about to graduate from high school, is an only child who was adopted at infancy by a single mother. Her relationship with her mother is characterized by symbiosis, anxiety about her condition, and over-protection. Meital, who was treated by the same arts therapist for three years, expressed anxiety in the sessions, as well as her challenges in dealing with day-to-day difficulties and distress at school. Her mother approached the arts therapist and asked for her help. The mother refused to go for private therapy because she claimed to have known the therapist for a long time, said she trusted her, and believed in her ability to help her and her daughter get through the crisis. Meetings were scheduled once a week, and at each meeting the next one was scheduled. There was no set timeframe for therapy in order to structure the therapy to be responsive to the needs of the mother and her daughter. During the parental guidance sessions with the mother, she expressed a great deal of anxiety about her daughter's eagerness to volunteer for the army, and about the transition from the safe and familiar framework of the school to an unknown framework and unpredictable future. The anxieties of both the mother and her daughter were processed in therapy and during sessions with the mother she learned to recognize her daughter's strengths, as well as her own when dealing with the transition from the school framework to the army. Meital became mentally stronger, began expressing her feelings in a more complete manner, recognized her abilities to cope and established separation and independence from her mother. This process of intervention during a crisis lasted several months with weekly therapy sessions between Meital and the arts therapist alongside meetings with the mother.

This model may not always be implementable. It requires commitment from the arts therapist, the parents, the support of the framework in which the arts therapist works and perseverance in the scheduled sessions, which is a challenge for arts therapists working in an educational-therapeutic program and for the parent to find the time to go to school. Despite these difficulties, the accessibility of therapy, its availability in the student's natural environment and the possibility of long-term therapy allow arts therapists to reach and engage students and parents and help them in the event of a crisis.

The third model describes the arts therapist's relationship with parents in parent-child groups in settings such as schools or treatment centers that provide services to the education system. The goals of these groups vary considerably (Kelly & Conture, 1991; McNeil et al., 1991; Niec, Hemme & Yopp, 2015) from providing information on mutual difficulties; for example, a group of parents and students with ADHD, or parents of children with behavioral problems. There are groups aimed at improving parent-child relationships by emphasizing optimal communication, as well as enhancing the parents' self-image, strengthening parental authority and helping parents guide and regulate their children's emotions. There are support groups for parents who share similar difficulties, which enable them to feel less alone, experience less shame and guilt and empower the parents and children. In some groups, parental guidance sessions are held separately, thus allowing parents to process their feelings, cope with difficulties and find adaptive and helpful ways of coping. These groups usually run for a short period of time between 10 to 12 sessions and typically meet in the afternoon or evening hours. There are also one-off topic-focused parents' groups that meet to provide information, lectures, sharing and the processing of subjects that are relevant to their children, such as adolescent development. These groups are led by arts therapists, psychologists and school counselors.

Summary and Conclusions

The importance of parent-child meetings as part of the therapeutic process is self-evident and necessary for processes of change to take place in the child and his/her parents. Various treatment approaches support this orientation, and some posit that when there is a lack of involvement of parents in the therapy provided to their children, there is no real therapy. The Israel Ministry of Education has examined the benefits of meetings between arts therapists and parents. The current recommendations mandate three meetings per year, at the beginning, middle and end of the year, and more if necessary. These recommendations are based on the consensus that these strong relationships help generate a more complete picture of what is going on in the child's life. The educational-therapeutic team receives detailed information from the parents and can assist and/or be assisted by them. Parents can also receive information about their child, get help in crisis situations and be involved and engaged in their child's therapy. These processes can enhance the relationship between the parties and the optimal acclimatization of the child as a result. However, maintaining the arts therapist-parent relationship is difficult. The factors that influence the relationship from the perspective of the arts therapist include the burden of a heavy caseload with a limited number of work hours that must incorporate meetings with parents, conflicting attitudes in the different work settings towards therapy, the seniority and experience of the arts therapist, his/her professional identity, therapeutic approaches and the perceptions of the parents. The factors affecting the relationship from the perspective of the parents include the financial loss of leaving work to attend meetings, difficulties identifying with the goals of the education system, their level of awareness of their child's difficulties, memories and experiences of their own childhoods in school, their anxiety about acknowledging and confronting their child's difficulties, fear of information disclosure and cultural barriers. Occasionally, there is an exceptionally low level of commitment to therapy to the extent of the complete absence of cooperation from parents, due in part to low socioeconomic backgrounds coupled with serious problems such as violence and the disintegration of the family structure.

Arts therapists find themselves in a dilemma in that their therapeutic approaches support and encourage meetings with parents, while the problematics of scheduling these meetings discourages it. In my opinion, it is important to arrange at least three meetings a year which are designed to gather information, help parents understand their child's difficulties, form a therapeutic alliance with the parents and collaborate and offer them support during the therapeutic process. Alongside the regular meetings during the year, specific models have been developed for exceptional circumstances when working with clients' parents. The first model, developed by Manor Binyamini (2014), focuses on the transitions children make in the education system: starting school, moving from grade to grade and to different school frameworks (elementary school, middle school, high school). The second model covers working with parents during times of crisis, and the third model involves parent-child groups that take place at schools or in treatment centers.

Schools now serve as more than basic educational institutions but also as settings attended by students with difficulties where they receive treatment. This underscores the need to maintain a regular meeting framework including the educational-therapeutic staff and parents. Currently in Israel three meetings with parents are held annually, but in order to adequately establish this relationship, the meetings should occur more frequently. The more the relationship between the arts therapist and the parents is clearly defined and institutionalized by the Ministry of Education, and supported by the allocation of hours and appropriate resources, the more significant the therapeutic process and changes will be, resulting in an increased level of cooperation between the parents and the educational-therapeutic staff. For these more frequent meetings to take place, the ratio of therapy hours to the number of clients should be redefined. In addition, therapists' work hours devoted to meetings, parental meetings, reports and supervision should be considered part of their paid workload.

The relationship between arts therapists and parents can also be strengthened by supervision and in-service education programs for arts therapists. Educating all the actors in the school system on the importance of collaboration and involvement of the parents is also crucial. The provision of supervision and continuing-education programs for arts therapists will generate a theoretical platform which is typically not acquired in professional training programs for arts therapists. During supervision, the arts therapists can explore case studies and learn ways of coping and working with parents.

Notes

1 The "therapist-parent relationship" is also commonly referred to as "parental guidance."
2 These examples are composites, and details have been masked to protect clients' privacy.
3 In most cases in the education system, only one parent attends these meetings, most often the mother.

References

Belity, I., Regev, D., & Snir, S. (2017). Supervisors' perceptions of art therapy in the Israeli education system. *International Journal of Art Therapy*, *22*(3), 96–105.

Bray, M. (2001). *Community partnerships in education: Dimensions, variations and implications*. Paris: Unesco.

Chethik, M. (2003). *Techniques of child therapy: Psychodynamic strategies*. New York: Guilford Press.

Cohen, E. (2006). "Parental level of awareness": An organizing scheme of parents' belief systems as a guide in parent therapy. In C. Wachs & L. Jacobs (Eds.), *Parent-focus child therapy: Attachment identification & reflective function* (pp. 39–64). New York: Rowman & Littlefield Publication.

Espasa, F.P. (2004). Parent–infant psychotherapy, the transition to parenthood and parental narcissism: Implications for treatment. *Journal of Child Psychotherapy*, *30*(2), 155–171.

Fonagy, P., Gergely, G., Jurist, J.E., & Target, M. (2002). *Affect regulation, mentalization, and the development of the self*. New York: Other Press.

Fraiberg, S. (1980). *Clinical studies in infant mental health*. New York: Basic Books.

Frick, P.J, Barry, C.T, & Bodin, S.D. (2000). Applying the concept of psychopathy to children: Implications for the assessment of antisociafl youth. In C.B. Gacono (Ed.), *The clinical and forensic assessment of psychopathy*. New York: Routledge.

Friedman, Y. (2011). Relations between the school and the parents in Israel. *Management and Education Organization Studies*, *32*, 237–267. (in Hebrew).

Green, C.L., Walker, J.M., Hoover-Dempsey, K.V., & Sandler, H.M. (2007). Parents' motivations for involvement in children's education: An empirical test of a theoretical model of parental involvement. *Journal of Educational Psychology*, *99*(3), 532.

Gutman, L.M., & Midgley, C. (2000). The role of protective factors in supporting the academic achievement of poor African American students during the middle school transition. *Journal of Youth and Adolescence*, *29*(2), 223–249.

Harris, A., & Goodall, J. (2008). Do parents know they matter? Engaging all parents in learning. *Educational Research*, *50*(3), 277–289.

Ishay-Karin, N. (2004). "Exposed in the frontline": Therapists' perceptions of parents. (in Hebrew). Retrieved from: https://www.hebpsy.net/me_article.asp?article=341

Kelly, E.M., & Conture, E.G. (1991, November). Intervention with school-age stutterers: A parent-child fluency group approach. In *Seminars in speech and language* (Vol. 12, No. 4, pp. 309–322). 1991 by Thieme Medical Publishers, Inc.

Lee, J.S., & Bowen, N.K. (2006). Parent involvement, cultural capital, and the achievement gap among elementary school children. *American Educational Research Journal*, *43*(2), 193–218.

Manor-Binyamini, I. (2014). Collaboration between parents of children with disabilities and professionals in schools. In *School-parent collaborations in indigenous communities* (pp. 93–135). New York: Springer.

McNeil, C.B., Eyberg, S., Hembree Eisenstadt, T., Newcomb, K., & Funderburk, B. (1991). Parent-child interaction therapy with behavior problem children: Generalization of treatment effects to the school setting. *Journal of Clinical Child and Adolescent Psychology*, *20*(2), 140–151.

Niec, L.N., Hemme, J.M., & Yopp, J.M., (2015). Parent-child interaction therapy: The rewards and challenges of a group format. *Cognitive and Behavioral Practice*, *12*, 113–125.

Nissimov-Nahum, E. (2008). A model for art therapy in educational settings with children who behave aggressively. *The Arts in Psychotherapy*, *35*(5), 341–348.

Regev, D., Snir, S. (2014). Working with parents in parent–child art psychotherapy. *The Arts in Psychotherapy*, *41*(5), 511–518.

Shamri-Zeevi, L. Regev, D., & Snir, S. (2015). Art- based interventions in the framework of parental training. *The Arts in Psychotherapy*, *45*, 56–63.

Shumow, L., & Miller, J.D. (2001). Parents' at-home and at-school academic involvement with young adolescents. *The Journal of Early Adolescence*, *21*(1), 68–91.

Snir, S., Regev, D., Keinan, V., Abd El Kader-Shahada, H., Salamey, A., Mekel, D., … Alkara, M. (2018). Art therapy in the Israeli education system–a qualitative meta-analysis. *International Journal of Art Therapy*, *23*(4), 169–179.

Wallace, M. (2013). High school teachers and African American parents: A (not so) collaborative effort to increase student success. *The High School Journal*, *96*(3), 195–208.

Winnicott, D.W. (1965). *The maturational processes and the facilitating environment*. London: The Hogarth Press and the Institute of Psycho-Analysis.

3 Maintaining Therapeutic Confidentiality in the School System

Nava Frieman

Introduction

Since my graduation in 2006, my work as a drama therapist and as a supervisor for students and arts therapists has involved maintaining confidentiality. This issue is an integral part of my daily work and raises many ethical and complex questions regarding many of my clients in the educational system. Other arts therapists have expressed similar concerns over the years.

Mutual sharing is a significant factor in my close and intensive work with the educational staff in schools. Our relationship is perceived as part of the systemic work of co-managing student issues and progress at school. Sharing is viewed as an advantage, a challenge and as a model by the staff and often by the arts therapists to achieve these students' educational and therapeutic goals. My personal experience has taught me that systemic work directed towards students in the school system often serves as an anchor for teachers and arts therapists by providing a space for joint consultation, thinking and dealing with difficulties together.

This feeling of togetherness can alleviate the sense of difficulty in situations where we as a team are required to deal with complexities that arise in work with students. At the same time, over the years I have experienced many difficulties working with the school staff, due to issues related to professional confidentiality, and respect for students' dignity and privacy. These situations raise ongoing dilemmas for both the staff and myself as to the best possible way to conduct ourselves during the information sharing process, so that it responds to the wishes and needs of each client to keep what occurs in therapy sessions confidential and prevent it from circulating outside the therapy room. However, I have often observed breaches of confidentiality that ultimately cause harm to the client in the school space, even though the initial intention was positive and was viewed as beneficial for the student.

This issue has prompted me to speculate and have doubts as to the nature of sharing and its implications. I have often noticed that sharing is carried out for unethical reasons and is followed by insensitive and careless conduct towards the students' private concerns. I have also noticed that in some cases, instances of sharing like these can jeopardize the client and the therapeutic process, as well as the student's trust in the teachers, the system and of course in me as a drama therapist. I have often felt that neither the team nor I had the proper tools to deal with these complex situations. At times, I have had feelings of confusion, guilt and sorrow as a result of situations in which, in retrospect, the client appeared to be badly affected by mutual information sharing, and the issue was perceived by the student as a breach of confidentiality and trust. I have wondered why my participation in student information sharing processes makes me feel negative, and by extension disappointed and unprofessional, such that these feelings continue to preoccupy me after exchanges with the staff. For these reasons, I decided to research this topic as part of the M.A. Program for experienced therapists in Drama Therapy at Tel Hai College, supervised by Prof. Sharon Snir. The findings are presented in this chapter.

Even before I began my research, I realized that as a drama therapist I initially felt committed to maintaining clients' privacy and confidentiality under the code of ethics for therapists and mental health professionals, but that on the other hand, systemic work often required me to deal with specific ethical dilemmas beyond those inherent to the therapist-client relationship that emanate from the nature of in-school therapy itself.

In various situations where I have had to deal with the systemic space regarding a client at school, I have not always been able to find a clear answer to the dilemma of confidentiality. I felt that the teaching staff and I did not share a common language of ethics and I often had to go through a complex decision-making process in which I did not always clearly understand whether the correct considerations were being made by the staff and myself, or whether they would harm or benefit the therapeutic process and/or systemic work. This situation led me to pursue a more in-depth examination of what was taking place in various schools regarding the protection and violation of confidentiality in the context of arts therapists. I sought to understand the causes that led to these situations in order to re-examine and tailor the ethical codes on confidentiality and generate more appropriate and up-to-date operational models for systemic conduct specific to schools in terms of maintaining confidentiality.

The chapter is based on interviews I conducted with arts therapists for research purposes on this topic, as well as my personal experience from the field. It presents the advantages, disadvantages and problems that arise during collaborative systemic work between arts therapists in the education system, as well as my work in the context of protecting confidentiality, preventing breaches, the ways we as therapists are currently attempting to address these situations, and suggestions for dealing with future challenges. I present examples reflective of many different clients treated over the years, which thus do not represent one specific client.

Theoretical Background

Arts therapists, by virtue of their work in the sensitive field of mental health, are required to adhere to a professional code of ethics which defines appropriate behavior in therapist-client and peer-to-peer relationships (American Psychological Association, 2019). This Code of Ethics primarily centers on therapists' responsibilities towards their clients, and their duty to put the clients' needs before those of personal interests. Of all these ethical obligations, confidentiality appears to be the most familiar, intuitive and widely accepted by both therapists and clients. Confidentiality is defined as therapists' ethical obligation to maintain confidential medical information disclosed during the therapeutic process. The prohibition against revealing client information is based on the client's right to privacy and on the principle that personal medical information belongs to the client (Corey, Corey, & Callahan, 1994).

However, this stipulation also appears to be the least well understood, and one that is difficult for therapists to implement and that many professionals violate (Bond & Mitchels, 2014). The ethical principles of respecting the independence and autonomy of the client, the right of the client to be treated justly, fairly and with loyalty, the right to privacy, to make decisions independently, to do good and avoid harm are the basic tenets governing confidentiality.

This ethical obligation is also crucial to the success of the therapeutic process. From the beginning, maintaining confidentiality encourages clients to seek out therapy despite their fear of social stigma. During the therapeutic process, ensuring confidentiality creates a sense of trust and confidence, forms the basis and strengthens therapeutic work (Bond & Mitchels, 2014). This pledge provides a space in which the client can trust the therapist and share his/her inner world and most private secrets, and gain a sense of openness and willingness to discover things about his/herself that were previously unknown or concealed due to anxiety, social prohibition or shame (Levin, Furlong, & O'Neill, 2003). This emotional content is critical during therapy and the ability to present the content in a safe and protected space provides an opportunity to treat such issues.

However, there are cases in which absolute confidentiality cannot be maintained despite these ethical obligations and the acknowledgment of its importance. Confidentiality is violated in cases where therapists are required by law to provide information to the authorities that they have acquired during therapy, for the benefit and well-being of the client and the public. Academic and/or professional objectives can also be reasons for information disclosure, provided that the identity of the client is concealed and non-identifiable (Donner, Vandecreek, Gonsiorek, & Fisher, 2008). In addition, each country has its own regulations for the psychotherapeutic professions specifying those conditions in which confidential information can be revealed, including situations in which the therapist believes that the disclosure of information is necessary for providing the best possible therapy for that client. Furthermore, this law often includes stipulations as to when therapists can provide information to other therapists for the purpose of treating the client. The laws and ethical rules in different countries were established to provide the therapist with directives to deal with various problems, but they do not always offer clear guidelines for specific cases, so that therapists are then called upon to exercise professional judgment. In reality, complex situations that raise ethical dilemmas can arise in the moral, legal and therapeutic domains and force the therapist to choose between different and occasionally conflicting values.

The issue of maintaining confidentiality is particularly challenging in systemic therapeutic work as found in educational systems. Arts therapy in schools is provided by an in-school arts therapist during school hours and gives students in the system who are dealing with emotional, developmental and learning difficulties and disabilities the therapy and support that will enable them to better cope with their role as students (Paternite, 2005). The arts therapist is given the opportunity to observe the client in his/her natural environment, and to interact with family and school staff (Regev, Green-Orlovich, & Snir, 2015). These advantages are coupled with a number of drawbacks. One of the key difficulties mentioned in the literature is the disparity between orientations with different and often contradictory languages such as the educational orientation and the therapeutic-dynamic orientation, which causes a variety of conflicts (Moriya, 2006), misunderstandings of the essence of therapeutic work and unmet expectations and requirements (Moriya, 2006; Nelson, 2010). The difference between these two orientations is also reflected in the way they perceive ethical standards, and this results in arts therapists having to deal with complex situations concerning client confidentiality and privacy (Jacob & Powers, 2009; Moriya, 2006; Randick & Dermer, 2013). In situations where conflicts of interest arise between the needs of the student and the needs of other parties (Lehr, Lehr, & Sumarah, 2007), arts therapists and researchers in the field recommend dealing with issues related to confidentiality based on a number of different factors, such as the child's age, level of emotional and cognitive functioning and the severity of the difficulties that the client faces (Bodenhorn, 2006; Lazowsky, 2008). Despite these recommendations, arts therapists are called upon to make complex choices regarding confidentiality partly due to the disparities and conflicts of interest between their personal and professional needs and the institutional needs of the school, which further exacerbates the situation by creating disputes over loyalty.

The challenges, difficulties and dilemmas that arts therapists face when working in the educational system are presented in the next sections in the context of maintaining confidentiality in systemic work. The aim is to define the needs that arise from these complex situations to suggest ethical, theoretical and operational standards and models for these dilemmas in schools which remain inadequately resolved.

Description of the Working Model and Clinical Examples

The research I carried out on this topic was based on interviews I conducted with ten arts therapists who have between 3 and 22 years of field experience. The arts therapists attended accredited universities or colleges in Israel and work in schools in different areas of the country. The objective was to examine arts therapists' perceptions on the issue of maintaining therapeutic confidentiality within the school setting. This work was prompted by an acknowledgment of the complexity of maintaining confidentiality in systemic work in schools, despite the importance of teamwork and the importance of sharing information about students. It was conducted to expand the theoretical scope on this subject, to better understand and analyze the complexities involved and to find solutions to improve the current situation.

When Should Information Emerging in Arts Therapy Be Made Available to Third Parties? The Need for a Gradual Process

According to the ethical codes of the therapeutic and medical professions, the therapist is obligated to report to the authorities when a client exhibits a genuine intention to commit a crime or cause harm to him/herself, to others or to property. This is also the case when the therapist suspects child abuse or neglect or when a court issues a warrant for such information (Carmichael, 2006; Moon, 2006). However, the way this rule is applied varies considerably such that in some cases it is unclear whether the duty of reporting applies to therapists.

Often I have found myself and my fellow school arts therapists colleagues debating the issues as to when we should share information disclosed in therapy to third parties, who should have access to this information and the appropriate method to convey it. In many cases when I felt the need to share information or the obligation to report information, I felt that for the benefit of the client and the therapeutic process, time was needed for consultation, deliberation or clarification with the client to have a clearer picture and choose the appropriate course of action.

In my research, one of the arts therapists described the dilemmas related to a student at risk with whom she worked. Some of the content that the student disclosed to her was conveyed outside the therapy room. It was not entirely clear to her whether this was a criminal case which she would be required to report. She decided to wait to report until she talked further with the client and consult with a psychologist and a colleague. After doing so, she realized that she was not obligated to report the issue. Thus, the postponement of reporting to external parties seems to be crucial in some cases.

Another similar case occurred when I was treating a child who was living with a foster family. The child's parents were divorced, and his mother was dealing with mental illness. The child told me that during his visits to his mother, men came to see her, touched her and took items from her room and that he felt unsafe. When he shared this with me, he asked me not to disclose this information outside of the therapy room because he feared that it would endanger his younger brother who has a severe syndrome and lives with his mother, and might be placed in foster care as well. From the beginning of the therapeutic process, we discussed the subject of confidentiality and because it was important for me to continue to allow him to feel a sense of security and trust in me, I tried to understand what the right thing would be to do before reporting the incident to minimize the expected consequences of disclosure. As a result, I consulted with the social worker as well as his school counselor and teacher in an attempt to make an appropriate decision for the student and manage the information disclosure process accordingly. The time I invested in consultation actually helped me as an arts therapist to feel safer and more accepting of the process that occurred at a later stage. It enabled me to share my concerns with the client about the exposure and my considerations which arose from the need to protect him in the precarious situation he was exposed to. It is worth noting that despite the gradual process of transmitting information from therapy to external parties, the client had feelings of intrusiveness and said that he was not yet ready for external intervention. He felt hurt and disappointed that I had disclosed information that he brought up in therapy. After disclosing the information, despite my attempts to act in the best interests of the client during the therapeutic process and when transmitting the information, I was still slightly disappointed with the outcome of the situation, since the client felt disappointed and uncertain, and it felt as though the therapeutic process had spiraled out of control. After the disclosure of information and the crisis that ensued, we had to process the complex events it entailed and its implications for our relationship. With all the complexities in this situation, the client continued to attend arts therapy, and we emerged from the crisis together. This case taught me that building trust within relationships, stating the limitations of confidentiality at the beginning of the therapeutic process, along with the gradual and slow process of disclosing information from therapy, allowed for the continuation of therapy following the crisis.

These cases emphasize the need for the arts therapist to reach understandings and arrive at decisions as to the best way to deal with the client at the various stages of disclosure. In my experience, there are situations where it is not possible to consciously manage this process in advance due to the complexity of the processes and the level of urgency of disclosure. However, in situations where this is possible and significant emotional content related to reporting can be processed, it is important for the arts therapist to be active in presenting the therapeutic information on these issues concerning confidentiality and during the stages of disclosure.

When the arts therapist understands clearly that the information disclosed in therapy needs to be reported, there is time to prepare the client before the reporting process. It is beneficial to explain the reasons why the therapist has decided to report information to the client. The therapist can describe his/her perceptions and feelings about the physical and/or mental dangers threatening the client, or those close to the client. The professional decision to disclose the information is made by the therapist; however, if the therapist shares his/her motivations with the client, as well as thoughts and feelings that led to this decision, this process may allow the client to feel part of the decision and somewhat in control of the situation and its unfolding. The preparation process is important because it may allow for processing of the client's fears of exposure and prepare him/her for future scenarios. Acknowledging and validating the content that will be reported, as well as allowing for the processing and containment of such content, are of immense importance.

During the exposure stage, it is important for the arts therapist to accompany the client in the processes that he/she is experiencing. Conscious and unconscious internal processes should be addressed when the client is confronted with the disclosure and clients should be made aware of the meaning and implications of these mental processes. This accompaniment stage enables the client to have curative experiences when dealing with feelings such as harm, danger, lack of control, helplessness and other feelings, which the client or someone close to the client may have experienced in the deleterious conditions that led to the reporting of information.

Once the information is disclosed, all the components of the process that took place must be processed. It is important to allow the client to examine how he/she perceived the experience of disclosure and its meaning, and to elaborate on the way the client thinks about and experiences it. The purpose is to allow the client to view the experience from an integrative perspective that can contain the aspects that he/she may perceive as adverse to the process of disclosure, and also those that embody the protection and support needed as a result of the disclosure. The very existence of the arts therapist and client's shared dialogue during these processes can strengthen the relationship, the therapeutic alliance and the level of trust.

The Arts Therapist Expresses the Need to Involve the Educational Staff

In cases where reporting is needed as well as those in which it is ultimately not necessary, many arts therapists, myself included, prefer to share information with the staff about the client's condition and the behavioral implications outside the arts therapy room. This is done to help the staff have a better grasp of the client's inappropriate behaviors outside of therapy and to provide help by establishing a support system for the client. In my experience, and consistent with the findings here in general, the need for the staff to participate in client-related matters also stems from the need for the involvement of other staff members, particularly the teacher, to uphold and contain the client's emotional content. In this way, the client's needs outside the arts therapy room can be met at a time when he/she needs the extra support, and the arts therapist can share the emotional burden with other professionals. In many instances where I shared my concerns with professionals outside the therapy room, I felt a sense of relief, less isolated in the process and more confident in the therapy process I was leading.

Staff members also approach the arts therapist often to ask for information about the client. This relationship is particularly true as regards the teacher. Even though such requests are based on a need to find an effective way to help the student and better understand how to deal with him/her, they generate many problems and areas of conflict. These situations have often evoked further feelings and confusion concerning my loyalties as an arts therapist; namely, whether I am being loyal to my client or unconsciously trying to live up to the staff's expectation as a co-worker by sharing meaningful information from the therapeutic process.

These dilemmas, which emerge in the context of breach of confidentiality in various situations, raise concerns not only for me but also for all other arts therapists who were interviewed in the study as to its negative impact in terms of the client's trust, the therapeutic process and the therapeutic alliance. The primary concern that emerged was that clients may suffer as a result of intrusive and ineffective interventions during the process of disclosure, feel uncertain about their sense of protection, and furthermore, the situation may cause the arts therapists to feel out of control concerning the clients' fate in the events following the disclosure process. These situations cause arts therapists to fear a negative impact on the therapeutic process. I often have these concerns because during the disclosure of the information or the subsequent process, when the information continues to be passed on to other parties such as other school staff or even welfare agencies, I occasionally feel that the benefit to the client is unclear and equivocal, and the transfer of information to external parties was carried out without considering the good of the client in terms of the factors involved, both by the individuals handing over as well as receiving the information. Therefore, arts therapists often fear that the harm that may be caused by the breach of confidentiality may outweigh the benefits to therapy. These concerns have often caused me and my colleagues many emotional difficulties in terms of failure to respect the clients' loyalty, privacy, rights and liberties.

A Lack of Awareness among Staff Members Results in a Breach of Confidentiality

A significant component of therapeutic work within the school system is the flow of communication between the educational staff and the arts therapist regarding clients while trying to maintain discretion. However, in many cases the educational staff reveal confidential material without being aware of doing so. The participants in the study also described similar situations in workplaces and events in the school space between different areas of the system.

Situations in which information related to arts therapy is transmitted indiscreetly may occur between teachers or staff members in a public place such as a staffroom or in the corridor. One example is a teacher's assistant who talks to the arts therapist aloud in the staffroom about a student who is disrupting class and whose behavior is so out of line that she does not want him to go on the annual school trip. This type of conversation in the staffroom can often turn into a public discussion about the student's behavior or background as different teachers mention their experiences with this challenging behavior.

Another example is when a teacher or staff member talks with a student inappropriately and in a non-discreet manner about information that the arts therapist disclosed. In these instances, the arts therapist assumed that the staff would not reveal this information to the student and would be able to use the information to better understand the student's behavior and adapt class interventions with this student accordingly. However, the unconscious behavior of the staff in these cases can generate heightened mistrust of the arts therapist and the therapeutic process on the part of the student.

An example of breach of confidentiality that resulted from a counselor's lack of awareness that was damaging to the client, the arts therapist and the therapeutic process was mentioned by one of the arts therapists in the study. The arts therapist described a case in which she reported to a counselor about a knife that a student from a special education class brought to school. She asked to go with the student to the counselor so that he could tell her about the knife in the presence of the arts therapist because the information came up during arts therapy and the arts therapist asked the counselor not to speak to the student without her. The counselor approached the student and told him that the arts therapist had told her that he possessed a knife, and then took him to the principal's office while yelling at him. The arts therapist stated in the interview that the event lasted a few seconds and was done in an unprofessional manner. The client noticed the arts therapist walking down the hall during this incident and shouted at her while others could see and hear, saying that she had betrayed him, she was a traitor and was on the police force. After this incident, the student refused to attend arts therapy for the rest of the year and undermined the arts therapist's professional status when he told everyone that she shared content from therapy and that she was a police officer. The arts therapist said that it took an entire month to get students to attend arts therapy because they were reluctant to see her.

Other cases that are indicative of teachers' lack of awareness of the need to maintain confidentiality occur during discussions between staff members and students about another student or client, or during discussions with students about their therapy process with the entire class. For example, a teacher asked the students in her class to share what was happening in their arts therapy sessions and what the arts therapist was doing during the sessions. Some students expressed dissatisfaction with their therapeutic process and with the arts therapist. As a result, one student expressed concern that he would not be able to continue therapy with his therapist because he feared that other students who were disappointed with their therapy would be referred to his arts therapist whom he perceived to be "good."

Other reasons for breaches of confidentiality caused by lack of awareness appear to be related to differences between the therapeutic and educational languages in systemic work. This gap often creates conflicts and a breeding ground for breaches of confidentiality by staff members. This can happen when students ask for help from the arts therapist to convey their difficulties to the teacher. Occasionally during these conversations, the teacher describes the students' inappropriate behavior to the arts therapist. The teacher, who usually perceives the arts therapist as part of the educational team, expects him/her to take the educational system's position towards the student, which does not always correspond to the arts therapist's therapeutic stance. For example, a client told the arts therapist about his feelings of stress and anxiety in class with a particular teacher because he felt that he did not understand the material and the teacher did not seem to notice what was wrong or help him. Feelings of stress and anxiety were portrayed in other situations that the client was experiencing. In this case, during the conversation with the arts therapist and given the client's needs to be seen and understood and because of his difficulty to meet with the teacher alone to express his feelings and needs, a suggestion was made to meet together with the arts therapist. The student and arts therapist hoped that the conversation would help the teacher address the student's distress during the lesson, both emotionally and practically, by devoting time to further explaining the material. In addition, the conversation was perceived as a therapeutic opportunity for the client to influence the situation and feel competent in the presence of the teacher.

During the conversation, the teacher explained how hard it was for her to deal with the emotional needs that the client and the arts therapist presented to her. The teacher focused on his "disruptive" behavior during class while describing to the arts therapist how his behavior interfered with the lessons, thus lowering the arts therapist's appraisal of the client. The arts therapist perceived the client's behavior as an expression of anxiety that he felt in situations of helplessness and frustration. The teacher asked the arts therapist in the presence of the student to help her explain to him how to behave appropriately in the classroom, which created a conflict with the student and reinforced his feelings that his needs had failed to be acknowledged yet again. This conflict reflects the gap between educational and therapeutic perceptions and demonstrates how a partial understanding of the therapeutic approach by the educational staff may result in a lack of discretion and unethical behavior in terms of maintaining confidentiality.

In my experience, ongoing and productive dialogue between the staff and the arts therapist as concerning clients' needs and difficulties in school, as well as the staff's uncertainty as to how to approach and address these clients, may be helpful in situations that are characterized by a lack of awareness. Continuous and discreet contact between the staff members and the arts therapists can allow for the expression of different positions, different considerations and the sharing of feasible solutions about situations where confidentiality dilemmas arise. This form of sharing can lead to the development of a shared educational and therapeutic language. Nevertheless, given the complex realities of time allocation and resources for this purpose, alongside the staff's lack of awareness of confidentiality ethics, the school staff may not have sufficient wherewithal to act professionally in this regard. My wish and that of many other arts therapists, as shown by the findings and the literature, is to continue trying to find appropriate and feasible ways to increase the staff's awareness of the ethics of confidentiality in situations where they are required to share information as part of their systemic work in the school setting.

In addition, I believe in the importance of creating training courses on ethics which can serve as a basis for raising and teaching awareness. The participants in these training courses should ideally include the team of teachers and arts therapists, who will learn about confidentiality, engage in and deal with different dilemmas while identifying a set of behaviors and operative ways to deal with real-life cases together. It should be mandatory for teachers and arts therapists to attend these courses before the start of the academic year, as well as throughout the year during their professional work in the field.

Disclosure of Information and Dilemmas Regarding Confidentiality Associated with the Presence of Arts Therapy within the School System

The provision of arts therapy within the school system can create other dilemmas. In the school system, which is part of the client's daily life, the other relationships that the arts therapist maintains on both a professional and social level with individuals whom the client also knows may create a situation of "multiplicity." This occurs when the arts therapist, for example, treats the client's siblings, children in the client's class, children whom the client knows from school or when the client is a child of one of the staff members. These relationships pose a challenge to the therapeutic relationship and the issue of trust that exists in the therapy room. An arts therapist presented an example of this type of difficulty encountered when treating two children from the same class. She described two boys who were in the same class and were both in arts therapy with her. They spent an afternoon together at one of their homes and the boy hosting his friend hit him, which caused much distress for the visiting friend. The victim's mother filed a complaint with the police which resulted in significant implications for both boys in terms of their emotional experiences and conduct at school. In arts therapy, the two boys, each in his own session, separately raised issues related to this event, as well as queries as to whether the arts therapist could work with them discreetly given that she was treating them both. The arts therapist said that this situation elicited different and complex feelings about each client, as well as a heightened sensitivity for maintaining a professional and neutral attitude towards each of them. The arts therapist spent a long time deliberating how to respond to each client when the other asked her questions about the other client and whether he had revealed things to her about their relationship. This raised concerns about the impact of what the other student was saying to the arts therapist.

Treating siblings also often elicits conflicts in terms of loyalty and the difficulty of maintaining each sibling's privacy from the other. Arts therapists describe cases where the educational staff referred siblings for arts therapy and it is often difficult to explain that treating only one sibling would be more beneficial for both clients and their family. A considerable number of arts therapists mentioned difficulties regarding the separation needed to treat two siblings within the same school.

By contrast, other arts therapists argued that there are situations where it is not possible to work according to the ethical rules of the therapeutic world outside the school. They claimed that treating two siblings at the same school is indeed justified for clients from low socioeconomic backgrounds who need therapy and cannot access therapy anywhere else than the school framework. Accordingly, this situation is perceived as the lesser of two evils when there is only one arts therapist in the school and therefore the issue of confidentiality for each sibling is particularly complex. The arts therapists described the precautions they take in this type of case to uphold the therapeutic boundaries of each therapy by preventing information from flowing from one therapy framework to the other.

Treating the children of staff members within the school setting also creates complications. In these cases, complex interactions may ensue between the staff member/parent and the arts therapist who is also a colleague. In these situations, the arts therapist may struggle to create the necessary separation with the colleague, since s/he is also required to relate to the colleague as the client's parent. This limits the intimacy and discretion required to treat a student within the education system.

Intra-system relationships in the context of therapeutic work are the source of many other dilemmas. For example, a request from the arts therapist to obtain information from one staff member about another staff member, or when a client presents information in therapy regarding abusive behavior by a staff member who is also a colleague pose challenges to confidentiality in arts therapy. In situations where arts therapists are asked to provide information about problematic or disturbing behavior by a coworker with whom they work, the respondents here described an inner conflict between their duty to provide the information as expected to help the system, and their need to remain loyal to their colleagues. For example, one of the arts therapists described a case in which the school counselor asked her to have a series of chats with a teacher to provide guidance on how to deal with the emotional and behavioral difficulties faced by the students in her class. During these exchanges the teacher disclosed personal information. Afterwards, the counselor asked to be informed about the content that emerged during the conversations. The arts therapist acknowledged her obligation to fulfill the counselor's request as a representative of the system and understood the rationale. However, the arts therapist felt compelled to maintain discretion with respect to the teacher who talked openly about personal issues. During their conversation, the arts therapist was careful not to give the counselor too many details by speaking in general terms and stating that she was working with the teacher on setting boundaries and providing the students a sense of warmth in the classroom.

The issue becomes even more complicated when the individual providing the problematic information about the staff member is a student being treated by the arts therapist. Clients often disclose information to the arts therapist during therapy and sometimes describe a teacher's hurtful behavior, such as disrespect, insults, a failure to listen and a misunderstanding of their needs, as well as the feeling that they cannot approach the teacher. Clients may describe their distress during arts therapy because they are upset and need help from the arts therapist. Several arts therapists stated that this situation raises many questions about the right course of action as to the information revealed during therapy and whether clients should be involved in these deliberations. On the one hand, they feel committed to the staff member as their colleague and are afraid to disclose the information that emerged during therapy because of the potential implications for their relationship with the staff member and the implications for their clients. However, they also described their sense of obligation to work towards improving their clients' emotional states. Ultimately, the arts therapists feel compelled to help students reveal information despite the considerations and concerns about the outcome of such disclosure. The preferred way to deal with such situations is to process the content with the clients during therapy so that the students can then feel free to report these circumstances to the school principal and to their parents. At the same time, arts therapists are aware of the damage that can be caused in any event of disclosure despite its importance to clients.

In situations described above, the system often exerts pressure on arts therapists to side with their needs, but as Moriya (2006) argued, arts therapists should set priorities and determine who is the dominant client. For example, in the case where the student complained about the arts therapist's colleague, the arts therapist decided that the student in therapy would take priority and acted accordingly. There may be situations in which arts therapists will not be able to fully identify and agree with the needs of the system, but it is important that they are able to take an empathetic approach to the needs of the system by expressing their professional position even if it runs counter that of the system.

Differences between Regular Education and Special Education in Terms of Maintaining Confidentiality

My work over many years in a special education school has made me appreciate attitudes and the professional orientation anchored within the system and in other special education schools, which was also mentioned by other arts therapists. This orientation is characterized by established and defined teamwork in the form of professional meetings about students which are attended by the educational and therapeutic staff for therapeutic and educational work. They discuss the dilemmas that arise in matters concerning confidentiality as part of their systemic work. In this way, a collaborative work process is established in which the staff members can communicate difficulties, examine the situation and the dilemmas and decide on professional and effective ways of dealing with ongoing dilemmas. This process allows for a clear definition and outline of ethical work codes that the staff accepts, which are the outcome of the mutual understanding and collaborative work that was carried out. The purpose of these discussions and consultations is to make the decisions that are the least damaging to client confidentiality.

Arts therapists working in regular school frameworks describe a different situation in which the staff are generally unavailable for collaboration or sharing information about the students. They also describe the struggle to allocate time for staff meetings and the scarcity of resources to support their therapeutic work. All these factors restrict the staff's ability to create norms to effectively deal with dilemmas concerning confidentiality. The staff meetings dealing with therapeutic issues do not take place often enough so that the staff and the arts therapists feel that they do not have the appropriate framework at work to discuss and consult about therapeutic issues, including that of confidentiality. It is important to build a collaborative and solid teamwork model in regular schools and from there establish appropriate ethical and therapeutic policies regarding students in terms of confidentiality.

Different Approaches to Ensure Confidentiality in Systemic Work

According to several arts therapists, and as I have found in my personal experience, the best way to deal with situations that engender dilemmas about transmitting information outside of therapy is to allow for a suitable thinking and therapeutic process to take place so that further actions can be taken after deliberation. From the start of the process that lays the groundwork for the therapeutic contract, it is important to emphasize the issue of building trust in therapy, which includes a discussion about confidentiality. This task may not be a simple one, since discussing the nature of confidentiality may on the one hand increase the client's confidence in the therapeutic process, but on the other may also threaten it (Moon, 2006). Nevertheless, this discussion right from the start of therapy may serve as an anchor if a breach of confidentiality arises. Therefore, it is important that at this stage the arts therapist adhere to the ethical rules of the therapeutic professions and emphasize his/her commitment to maintaining confidentiality, but also the limitations involved to the client. This is of particular importance in schools where daily reality is often part of the therapeutic situation.

During the process of establishing the therapeutic contract, I recommend that the arts therapist emphasize to the student that in case a decision needs to be made regarding a breach of confidentiality (Corey et al., 1994), confidentiality issues will be brought to the arts therapy room in a therapeutic manner. They will be discussed in the context of the therapist-client relationship while sharing the various considerations and the meaning and the purpose of disclosing information to outside parties with the client. It is preferable for the arts therapist to attempt as much as possible to obtain the client's consent for the decisions being made (Corey et al., 1994; Moriya, 2006). In this way, informing the client about the limitations of maintaining confidentiality from the start of the process can help uphold the trusting relationship even after the arts therapist relays information or reports on an issue that necessitates disclosure. The more accurately the information is presented by the arts therapist to the client at the beginning of the process, the less problematic the client's emotional response in these situations will be and a process can take place that achieves the desired results for both the client and his/her environment. Furthermore, if and when it occurs, the breach of confidentiality can then be addressed without causing irreversible damage to the therapeutic alliance and in a way that can protect the client without the breach of confidentiality being perceived as hostile but rather as an act motivated by genuine concern (Hass & Malouf, 2002).

In doing so, the principles of doing good and maintaining respect for the client's autonomy are preserved while the rules of society are maintained. When a breach of confidentiality or sharing of information is required as part of the systemic work at the school for the benefit of the client (Essex, Frostig, & Hertz, 1996; Moriya, 2006), it is important for the arts therapist to maintain the client's privacy as much as possible during the process of information sharing, to share as little information as possible and to do so in a way that causes the least possible harm. These coping methods, when applied by arts therapists in the field, provide a space to exercise professional judgment and make decisions based on freedom of choice and a sense of responsibility. Underlying this approach is the concept that the cornerstone of therapy is trust and not absolute confidentiality (Corey et al., 1994; Moriya, 2006).

Another key tool available to arts therapists when they are required to make decisions in difficult situations where the ethical or legal solutions are unclear and unequivocal are supervision sessions from other professionals in the field. Supervision has often helped me to understand how I want to proceed in certain dilemmas regarding confidentiality, and I try to offer the same guidance to arts therapists and students who come to me for supervision. In these situations, addressing the problem and the ability to approach it from different angles, which can only be carried out by someone who is not directly involved to allow for a process of evaluation, can lead to more appropriate behavior and avert errors and harm as much as possible. I am hopeful that arts therapists in the education system (myself included) will allow ourselves to view our professional efforts in these complex dilemmas in the context of confidentiality as a "good enough" effort to cope, and perceive this as a situation where we tried to do everything in our power to reach the best moral decision for us as arts therapists.

Summary and Conclusions

This chapter described the dilemmas that arts therapists face in terms of confidentiality in the school setting. A number of recommendations can be made. Given the many dilemmas and conflicts that arise around the issue of confidentiality, there seems to be room for realignment within the school system. It is crucial to base these efforts on ethical standards applied to models accepted by the therapeutic systems, where information is shared as needed with all individuals working with the student in therapy, and where the ethical rules of confidentiality have been designed for this purpose. The aim of collaboration and sharing of information is thus to help mediate the students' inner world to the staff and enable them to realize their abilities to fulfill key developmental tasks in school and especially as students. Many arts therapists have suggested that such a model should be initiated through ongoing work by individuals who specialize in issues such as ethics and confidentiality within the educational system as well as in the arts therapies field.

In addition, it is advisable to train the educational and therapeutic staff through confidentiality workshops and lectures which would help close the gap between the therapeutic and educational languages and establish a common code of ethical conduct in the school space with the client and in terms of the information transmitted between staff members about the client. Exposing the staff to dilemmas related to confidentiality, while studying the issue and discussing the various factors that emerge in this context, could serve as a basis for further understanding and internalization of the most appropriate ways to deal with these situations. In this way, arts therapists and educational staff can work together towards the common goal of student development. The arts therapists also suggested the continuation of training by professional supervisors to deal with the complexities of maintaining confidentiality in the school system and to support practice in the field.

This chapter, in the context of my research, examined the difficulties and conflicts faced by arts therapists when faced with issues related to maintaining and violating confidentiality as part of systemic work in the school setting. These conflicts oppose the value of sharing information regarding the student, which is based on the accepted view in schools that sharing information can often benefit the student, and the value of maintaining confidentiality, a fundamental and central tenet of therapeutic ethics.

I hope that the voices of the arts therapists from the field will raise awareness of the need for the creation of renewed and improved operative models of conduct in the therapeutic-educational space in the school, which is very different from the therapeutic environment that exists outside the school. Incorporating these future theories and models into training programs for arts therapists, counselors and teachers before entering the educational system, as well as during their employment, may help maintain client confidentiality in arts therapy within the systemic work in the school, and make it more effective and professional for the client.

References

American Psychological Association (2019). *Ethical principles of psychologists and code of conduct*. Retrieved from: https://www.apa.org/ethics/code

Bodenhorn, N. (2006). Exploratory study of common and challenging ethical dilemmas experienced by professional school counselors. *Professional School Counseling*, *10*, 195–202.

Bond, T., & Mitchels, B. (2014). *Confidentiality & record keeping in counselling and psychotherapy* (2nd ed.). London: Sage.

Carmichael, K.D. (2006). Legal and ethical issues in play therapy. *International Journal of Play Therapy*, *15*(2), 83–99. doi:10.1037/h0088916

Corey, G., Corey M., & Callahan, P. (1994). *Issues and ethics in the helping professions* (4th ed.). Pacific Grove, CA: Brooks/Cole.

Donner, M.B., Vandecreek, L., Gonsiorek, J.C., & Fisher, C.B. (2008). Balancing confidentiality: Protecting privacy and protecting the public. *Professional Psychology: Research and Practice*, *39*, 369–376.

Essex, M., Frostig, K.J., & Hertz, J. (1996). In the service of children: Art and expressive therapies in public schools. *Art Therapy: Journal of the American Art Therapy Association*, *13*(3), 23–27. doi:10.1080/07421656.1996.10759218

Hass, L.J., & Malouf, J.L. (Eds.). (2002). *Keeping up the good work: A practitioner's guide to mental health ethics* (3rd ed.). Sarasota, FL: Professional Resource Press.

Jacob, S., & Powers, K.E. (2009). Privileged communication in the school psychologist-client relationship. *Psychology in the Schools*, *46*, 307–318. doi:10.1002/pits.20377

Lazovsky, R. (2008). Maintaining confidentiality with minors: Dilemmas of school counselors. *Professional School Counseling*, *11*, 335–346.

Lehr, R., Lehr, A., & Sumarah, J. (2007). Confidentiality and informed consent: School counsellors' perceptions of ethical practices. *Canadian Journal of Counselling*, *41*, 16–30.

Levin, C., Furlong, A., & O'Neill, M.K. (Eds.). (2003). *Confidentiality: Ethical perspectives and clinical dilemmas*. Hillsdale, NJ: Analytic Press.

Moon, B.L. (2006). *Ethical issues in art therapy*. Springfield, IL: Charles C. Thomas.

Moriya, D. (2006). Ethical issues in school art therapy. *Art Therapy: Journal of the American Art Therapy Association*, *23*(2), 59–65.

Nelson, C.L. (2010). Meeting the needs of urban students: Creative arts therapy in Jersey City public schools. *Art Therapy*, *27*, 62–68.

Paternite, C. (2005). School-based mental health programs and services: Overview and introduction to the special issue. *Journal of Abnormal Child Psychology*, *33*, 657–663. doi:10.1007/s10802-005-7645-3

Randick, N., & Dermer, S. (2013). The relationship of school art therapy and the American School Counselor National Model. *Art Therapy*, *30*(1), 30–35. doi:10.1080/07421656.2013.757507

Regev, D., Green-Orlovich, A., & Snir, S. (2015, September). Art therapy in schools – the therapist's perspective. *Arts in Psychotherapy*, *45*, 47–55. doi:10.1016/j.aip.2015.07.004

4 The Integration of the Arts Therapies in the Work of a Multidisciplinary Team in a Hospital School Setting

Michal Ulitzur-Zemel, Yael Kalfus, Tal Mann and Haggai Yoel

Introduction

Alyn Hospital, a pediatric and adolescent rehabilitation center, is a unique national treatment center in Israel that specializes in the diagnosis and rehabilitation of children and adolescents with a variety of congenital and acquired physical disabilities. The center operates several departments including Pediatric Rehabilitation, Pediatric Respiratory Rehabilitation, Day Hospitalization Rehabilitation, an Outpatient Clinic, a Skills Development Center, a Therapeutic Sports Center, an Independent Living Neighborhood, a wing for Ventilator-Assisted individuals and a Rehabilitation Educational and Medical Day Care facility which has its own pre-schools, school and rehabilitation day care.

The school is integrated into Alyn's medical-rehabilitation structure. It is supervised by the Department of Special Education, which is regulated by the Ministry of Education and has two educational systems. The first consists of six classrooms serving six to ten children each. The students range in age from 3 to 21 and come from a variety of Jewish and Arabic, religious and secular, backgrounds. They have severe physical disabilities, congenital or acquired heart defects, neurological impairments (cerebral palsy, spina bifida), brain injuries, respiratory lung diseases that require artificial respiration, various traumatic injuries (some were injured in military or terror attacks), metabolic disorders and various other syndromes, some of which include intellectual disabilities. Most have language impairments of varying severity. Some of the students reside in the hospital boarding school, whereas others travel to school daily by shuttle bus. The second system has two classrooms designed for specific students who are admitted to the hospital's rehabilitation department, and others who are admitted to the day care facility. It serves approximately 30 students who have various traumatic injuries.

The therapeutic work is split into individual and group sessions and is integrated into the school framework during the morning hours as part of each class schedule. Each therapist has a dedicated workspace consisting of an art therapy room, a music therapy room and a therapeutic petting zoo located in an inner courtyard adjacent to the school. Each class convenes as a group with each therapist on a weekly basis and some students also receive individual therapy sessions.

Arts therapies are relatively new at Alyn Hospital and have only been operating in this setting since 2012. The team of arts therapists and animal-assisted therapists at Alyn were originally part of the educational staff. The transition from a teaching profession to a therapeutic profession and the establishment of an arts therapies and animal-assisted therapy space within the school was gradual and required a realignment of goals and expectations on the part of the therapists and the system at large. Art and music teaching hours transitioned into therapy hours, and early career therapists were given the task of shaping their new professional identity while at the same time paving the way and consolidating the status and position of arts and animal-assisted therapies within a larger system with unique, complex and challenging characteristics.

Theoretical Background

The key feature of the model presented in this chapter is the location of the school within a rehabilitative hospital. This means that the hospital staff includes professionals from the fields of education, medicine, mental health, nursing and rehabilitation. In addition to the classroom schedule, each student has a personalized work plan tailored to his/her individual needs, which includes healthcare treatment sessions such as physiotherapy, hydrotherapy, occupational therapy, speech therapy, arts therapies and animal-assisted therapy. The diverse array of professionals allows for a broad and comprehensive observation of each client but may also lead to disagreements between professionals. The issue of multiple treatments and the interactions between professionals tends to come to the fore when students are treated by both the arts therapists and the school psychiatrist or psychologist, and when each class receives group therapy from all of these therapeutic disciplines simultaneously. This complex situation requires the therapists to coordinate their goals and collaborate with a broad multidisciplinary team who work with these students and observe and assess them from different standpoints.

The students are typically divided into classes according to age, mother tongue and level of functioning. However, due to the small number of classrooms and the diverse characteristics of the students at Alyn Hospital, each class is made up of students with different levels of physical and mental functioning. Over and above their physical difficulties, some of them also have developmental disabilities, such as learning and language impairments. The educational and therapeutic programs thus need to be adapted to students with physical and developmental disabilities as well as to heterogeneous classes in which students at different levels of cognitive functioning study together.

In contrast to other hospitals where the length of hospitalization is usually time-bound and disrupts their normal routine, for most patients at Alyn Hospital their stay is part of their regular life. Some have lived in the hospital since they were born and others have come in daily for years. These patients in particular have movement, breathing and swallowing disabilities. Some are completely dependent on a respirator for breathing, whereas others are dependent on feeding tubes. Most have mobility difficulties and use wheelchairs and walkers, and some have limited verbal abilities and rely on alternative forms of communication. As a result, arts and animal-assisted therapists need to find creative methods to work with these young students who have limited access to the outside world and restricted movement abilities.

Art, music and animal-assisted therapies are particularly well-suited for the population at Alyn Hospital because they allow these students to better cope with the complex dialectic between health and illness which is intrinsic to a school operating within a hospital setting. They do so by creating a transitional space between the inner and outer worlds where the creative self can function and play (Winnicott, 1971). In these therapy sessions, the students can join in and participate as a function of their abilities. The art media also acts as another important channel of communication and self-expression that bypasses the structures of language and words. Arts and animal-assisted therapies contribute uniquely to the lives of the students admitted to Alyn Hospital because they utilize therapeutic methods in which the client is active and involved not only emotionally, but through movement, the use of the senses and cognition. Research suggests that these therapeutic methods contribute significantly to reducing stress and anxiety (Curry & Kasser, 2005), provide a distraction from pain and suffering (Nainis et al., 2006), enhance feelings of competence and self-worth and enhance individual coping skills (Favara-Scacco, Smirne, Schiliro, & Di Cataldo, 2001). The process of creativity and expression is an active one, and as such it is experienced as a "work of hope" (Hazut & Segev-Shoham, 2002) in that it encourages the client to initiate, make changes and find solutions, and promotes a sense of control, competence and independence (Malchiodi, 1999).

These students' complicated medical conditions necessitate accessible facilities and technical adjustments. All the classrooms are situated on the same floor, with a nurses' station in the center. The dedicated therapy rooms and the therapeutic petting zoo are also located on this floor. There is a limited number of children in each class, and there are several staff members present in every classroom at any given moment. The children in the classrooms mostly remain in stationary positions, either sitting or lying down next to their medical and rehabilitative devices while the staff members move between them. In addition to the regular staff in the classroom, the nursing staff go in and out of the classrooms regularly to provide critical physical care and monitor the students' physiological indicators. Thus, during group therapy sessions in the classroom, other staff members can also be present in the room. Hence, external factors pervade the therapeutic process and the therapists need to deal with disruptions to the regular therapeutic setting while striving to create a supportive, organized and containing environment (Bion, 2004; Winnicott, 1971); i.e., the experience of being surrounded by a protective and embracing skin (Anzieu, 2016), and provide a secure base (Bowlby, 1990) for development and growth.

During the sessions with each student, to provide an appropriate emotional response the therapists must take a wide range of individual mind-body information into account that influences the client's functioning and needs. The students' ongoing medical conditions have critical implications for their mental development. Most students, some from birth, have coped with ongoing or permanent separation from their parents, undergo recurrent and invasive medical procedures that cause discomfort, pain, distress and anxiety, as well as a loss of a sense of control or a complete lack of control, and some face the constant threat of death (Malchiodi, 1999). It can be assumed that their continued dependence on the medical staff and medical devices directly impacts these students' sense of separateness, differentiation, autonomy and self-efficacy; the recurrent stress and anxiety also reduce their feelings of security and mental well-being.

These students' precarious health conditions have implications for their immediate circle of classmates as well. These distressing situations are often reflected and resonate in their classmates' gazes and reactions. Some students at Alyn Hospital are constantly at risk of death and some unfortunately pass away at a very young age. Occasionally students witness the deterioration of a classmate and are forced to deal with his/her loss. Encountering the death of classmates is burdensome and difficult, and in the past the educational staff lacked the appropriate tools to cope with this reality. To palliate this need, the arts therapy team was asked to develop a new channel for coping with this issue, both for the students and the staff.

The therapists themselves encounter severe illnesses, pain and loss, and as a result may feel helpless and are at risk of burnout, secondary traumatization and compassion fatigue. In order to contain their clients, the therapists also need to be contained and held within a supportive framework that helps them maintain their strength, process countertransference, offer emotional support and clarify professional matters.

Another critical factor is the multicultural composition of the Alyn framework. The hospital setting creates an opportunity to break down barriers between the different sectors and social groups in Israel and connect them directly. The students and staff members are Jewish, Christian and Muslim from religious and secular backgrounds who have diverse opinions and worldviews and reside in a country characterized by a politically charged and fragmented reality (Bruno and Massarwa discuss this issue in detail in the next chapter). The day-to-day school setting can generate complex situations that require careful consideration of how to address traditions, beliefs, values and national heritage, as well as direct and indirect responses to the political situation and military events in the country and the region affecting both the staff and the students.

The reality that half of the children at Alyn Hospital speak Arabic but the arts and animal-assisted therapy staff are Hebrew speakers with only a basic knowledge of the Arabic language also has a direct effect on the verbal component of communication during therapy. Other staff members are present in the room to assist the therapists with Arabic translation during group sessions. The presence of a third party in the therapeutic space, as well as the actual need to translate emotional expressions through an intermediary, have profound implications for the dynamic in the therapy room, and raise professional and ethical questions that will not be addressed in this chapter, but are certainly worthy of mention and further examination. In individual therapy sessions, the therapists typically refrain from the inclusion of a translator, thus relinquishing the opportunity for mother-tongue expression and communication with the client.

Description of the Working Model and Clinical Examples

The special nature of the framework in which the arts and animal-assisted therapists work at Alyn Hospital calls upon them to deal with the complex conflict between internal and external content that can impede the creation of a therapeutic space in the classroom. Nevertheless, the therapy staff believe that art, music and animal-assisted therapy can contribute significantly to the students' quality of life since with flexible and creative thinking the unique characteristics of the setting can be harnessed to enable effective work. They also believe that the integration of arts and animal-assisted therapies at Alyn Hospital does not only present a challenge but can bridge the gap between different languages and spaces.

The features of the therapeutic setting at this school prompted the team of arts and animal-assisted therapists to create a holistic working model to respond to emotional, social and community goals. The arts and animal-assisted therapies at Alyn Hospital aim to create a transitional space that allows for the transition between the inner and outer worlds, form a bridge between the individual and the group, between language and cultural divergencies and between the severe physical limitations and the healthy functioning parts of each individual. The overarching goal is to contain and sustain the duality of health and illness, which is the key to the healing power and the ability to foster hope of these therapies.

The arts and animal-assisted therapists' therapeutic approach is well suited to the hospital's primary therapeutic objective of the rehabilitation of children and teens and the provision of assistance to support better functioning. Therefore, the therapeutic working model centers around expression and support. The purpose of the therapeutic process is to create a safe, containing and supportive space, provide an opportunity for exploration and experimentation, relief and relaxation, the expression of internal emotional content, the expression of each student's individuality and to enhance their sense of ability and self-worth. The core of the therapeutic work involves class groups since these sessions enable social learning, support and mutual feedback. Group therapy encourages interpersonal engagement, cooperation and social interactions between the students, awareness, their acknowledgment and sensitivity towards others, a sense of belonging and cohesion within the group, and the discovery of collective and shared issues among all group members. The working model at Alyn Hospital emerged from the facility's defined mission. The model takes a holistic approach which relates to the client as a complete individual so that all physical, mental, emotional and social needs are met. The therapeutic space has clear yet flexible boundaries that allow for both separation and accessibility simultaneously.

The arts therapists work as part of the multidisciplinary team and strive to obtain maximal information about the level of each student's medical, rehabilitative, educational, social, emotional and family-related functioning. Although their work focuses on the emotional components, it is conducted with an awareness of the goals and processes of other treatment plans. The working model is based on the view that the encounters between the different systems involved in these students' health and well-being constitute an advantage and opportunity for teamwork and collaboration. The working model emphasizes collaborations and connections. It focuses on creating a space for discourse and sharing between the individual and the group, between professionals from different fields, between the interior and the exterior and between cultures. The pivotal tool for creating this space is the arts. The model views the challenges inherent to the system as opportunities for initiative and growth.

A Space for Collaboration

The working model at Alyn Hospital is based on the idea of the creation of a space for collaboration between the different therapists, the therapists and other professional staff, and the therapists and parents. The shared daily presence of art and music therapists at Alyn Hospital almost every day of the week facilitates a continuous and effective dialogue between the various partners.

Collaboration within the therapeutic team. It is important for the therapeutic team to collaborate and coordinate their work because their group therapy sessions take place in the same classrooms. The structure of the group sessions required modifications in the overall class schedule to allow for routine group supervision and staff meetings, and for each of the therapists to work in each class on a different day of the week. The staff meetings are planned on a weekly basis with the educational staff and are used to formulate collaborative work plans around common goals or content that each of the therapists works towards within the framework of his/her profession. The weekly supervision session acts as an anchor and framework for emotional support and clarification of professional issues.

Collaboration with the educational team. The educational staff is typically not present during the therapy sessions. This means there must be continual updating and coordination with the therapy team. To do so, the arts therapy team holds a weekly meeting with the educational staff during their work hours where the teachers discuss topics and content that arise in their classes, as well as issues concerning the social and emotional state of each student. The therapists present their perspectives on the classroom and the students and use information from the teachers to adjust their therapeutic goals. The art and music therapists' previous work as teachers in the educational field gives them experience in engaging and discussing issues with the educational staff and also contributes to the level of cooperation and support between them.

For example, during one of the staff meetings, a teacher talked about a problem she had with two students. When she worked with the students individually, they showed they had understood the material, but when they were in the classroom, they were afraid of making mistakes and would not participate in class. Yael Kalfus, the arts therapist, suggested she would work on mistakes in her art therapy sessions. She presented the book "Beautiful Oops" (Saltzberg, 2010) to the class which describes a "mistake" on each page such as spilled gouache paints and crumpled paper, and how to make something new from each: the stain becomes a painting, the crumpled paper turns into a fuzzy sheep and so on. The students were excited about the creative ideas in the book and were then asked to experiment. Each chose a "mistake" from the art materials and turned it into a new artwork. Yael noticed that the new possibilities surprised them and enabled them to view a "mistake" from a new perspective. After the session, the students felt more relaxed and began to actively participate in classroom activities.

In another case, the teacher of the senior class asked the therapy team to help her develop and expand her students' emotional vocabulary. The discussion between the teacher and the therapists led to the joint creation of a learning curriculum which integrates the arts and aims to develop emotional language and a concomitant development of self-awareness. Yael, the arts therapist, together with the teacher, devised a lesson plan in which stories and pictures were presented to the students in the classroom. These facilitated conversations about emotions and at a later stage led to creative work. The teachers and teaching assistants actively participated in these activities and presented personal examples of emotional sharing and containment. An activity using the book "Silly Billy" (Browne, 2006) allowed the students to talk about their fears and then make worry dolls. The book "Room on the Broom" (Donaldson & Scheffler, 2016) was used to shift the conversation to the subject of surprises. The students noted the various surprises that appeared on the witch's path and spoke about their personal surprises. The class prepared boxes and each student picked a box and created a character that would pop out of the box by surprise. Before Tu BiShvat (a Jewish holiday; the New Year of the Trees), the students prepared a forest of emotions, and each student made a tree that represented one emotion such as a happy tree, a disappointed tree, a longing tree and so on. These activities gave the students and teachers an opportunity to discuss emotions in the classroom.

Tal Mann, the music therapist, organized combined meetings in the classrooms for students and the educational staff to provide the staff with ways to engage in emotional conversations with the students. Each session started with a routine where Tal strummed on the guitar, sang a song and addressed each student by asking how he or she was feeling. All the students were given the opportunity to play their feelings on the guitar, pick a card from the stack of emotion cards beside it and share their choice of emotion with the class. The students became accustomed to this morning ritual in which each of them was given the opportunity to express their emotions verbally and through music. The ritual helped them practice their listening skills and listen to each other patiently, and to enjoy being listened to. For some, the experience of being the center of attention was unfamiliar and often stressful. For many it was a chance to reveal themselves to others gradually and develop the ability to speak and share things with their friends and staff. After many years of this routine, the students' progress has been striking. At the start, the morning routine was relatively short and the students used few words to express themselves in a concrete manner. Over time, the students' vocabulary has expanded and their willingness to share has grown. At first, some of the students imitated each other and articulated the same emotions, but over time, and with the development of their empathic abilities, their capacity for self-expression has improved. This process has helped these students develop a sense of differentiation and find their true authentic selves. At a later stage, the themes formed the basis for inventing group songs, or alternatively one student would choose a song with the same theme and play it to the group. For example, one of the themes that emerged was rebellion; i.e., "I don't want to!" This theme emerged when one student revealed that he did not want to take a blood test because it hurt. Another student said he did not like his physical therapy because it was hard for him. A conversation arose in the classroom about how hard it is to undergo unpleasant medical and therapeutic interventions, while also recognizing their importance to their health. Drumming on drums helped the students release their anger as they yelled, "I don't want to!" Gradually the tension dissipated, and the expressions of anger progressively became moments of laughter and enjoyment. Tal played the song "I Don't Want" (by Noga Geva) and after the students learned the words, they asked to hear it played in the following sessions. The song became their theme song that related to everything they had to do but did not want to do, and created a channel for dialogue between the students and the multidisciplinary team. The students were given a tool to directly express their difficulties and oppositions, and the team was able to validate and contain these situations and negotiate with the students as to how different activities and procedures would be performed. The musical expression helped reduce the level of tension between the parties.

Another issue that arose was the theme of missing a sick classmate who had been absent from school for a long time. One student strummed gently on the guitar and shared his longing with the class. Then more students expressed their longing for the same classmate, and the class composed a song together with the therapist, each writing one line of the lyrics. The song was recorded, and they were pleased to learn that it would be played to their friend upon his return. The presence of the educational staff in these sessions fostered a better level of understanding on their part and more empathy towards the students' emotional worlds. It also significantly contributed to a more accepting and containing atmosphere in the classroom and provided the educational team with techniques for discussions about emotions which they could then apply daily in their work.

Collaboration with the paramedical team. The professionals who interact with the students at Alyn Hospital make it possible to provide integrated therapy. The arts therapists are cognizant of the medical-rehabilitative goals and can contribute directly or indirectly towards achieving them. Tal Mann, the music therapist, works in the rehabilitation day-care facility with the physical and occupational therapists. The music accompanies, supports and reiterates the motor-sensory exercises and helps reduce levels of stress and resistance. In the case study described below by Tal Mann, the emotional work also affected the physical aspects of the rehabilitation process. A 16-year-old boy suffered a head injury in a car accident. He was left with weakness in the left side of his body and speech difficulties. His parents described him as a talented and creative boy, loved by his family and friends and deeply connected to music. When the boy entered the music room for the first time accompanied by his father and some friends, he was brought inside in a wheelchair by his friend. The therapist could not see his face because he was bending over. Those accompanying him offered to remain in the room and sing his favorite songs. While listening to them, Tal observed the boy's reaction. His body remained bent over, but she noticed that he was gently tapping his foot on the floor to the music. She realized that he had shared the experience with them. The boy continued to attend weekly sessions. During the initial sessions, he was interested in small instruments such as wind chimes and drums, which raised his upper left body and put him in a position to look forward. As the sessions progressed, he began to sit up straight and later, when he was already sitting upright, he began to take an interest in the larger instruments that were suddenly visible to him and chose to play the set of drums. It was very important for him to play with both hands at a consistent pace to produce a "good sound," which was impressive and required him to make a great deal of effort. As he drummed, whether out of a love of music or to "make it sound like it should," the therapist realized that he was unintentionally repeating his physical therapy exercises over time and with considerable effort, thus strengthening his weak hand. He later discovered the piano and began to compose songs. Some of the songs started from lyrics that he wrote, and others began with a tune he discovered while improvising on the piano. At the outset, he only played with his right hand, his healthy hand. When he felt that one of the songs was almost ready, he would add a musical accompaniment with his left hand. The music therapist was astounded by his effort to play with his weak hand, which could barely be lifted into position at the piano and required him to move each finger separately. This was a successful rehabilitative task for his occupational therapy exercises. He spent many sessions composing appropriate musical accompaniments for his songs. He also expressed the desire to sing while playing with both hands. Initially he sang monotonously and slowly, but his insistence on the quality of the performance prompted his speech therapist to take part in several sessions specifically dedicated to voice production and training. The content of the songs directly expressed the boy's effort to produce the songs and deal with the rehabilitation process. The boy recovered and today functions independently. He continues to compose songs and play music, and recently returned to Alyn Hospital as a volunteer.

Collaboration with the parents. Some parents stay in the rehabilitation department with their hospitalized children, go with them to treatment and occasionally even stay with them during the therapy sessions because of the child's physical or emotional dependence on them. Despite this complexity, the parent's presence gives therapists the opportunity to observe the parent-child relationship and exchanges. It also provides an opportunity for family interventions and parent-child therapy sessions which can promote growth and change. The following case study shows how the presence of a mother alongside her three-year-old daughter contributed towards and promoted the therapeutic process.

Ayala (pseudonym), who was born approximately a year after her family immigrated to Israel, has a severe degenerative disease. She cannot move independently other than slight movements of her limbs, she breathes with a respirator and is fed through a feeding tube. In her first year at Alyn, Ayala did not speak, was grim and communicated with the staff solely through eye movements. When she wanted to say yes, she closed her eyes, and to respond no she rolled her eyes up. During the sessions with her parents, the staff learned that there was a significant gap between her level of communication at home and at school. At home she felt more at ease and spoke freely and fluently. Ayala was diagnosed with selective mutism, and it was decided that all the staff members who worked with her would focus on establishing a relationship of trust, and temporarily set aside any other rehabilitation goals. Despite her basic trust in her music therapist,

Ayala did not speak during the sessions. Concurrently, most of the songs that she chose were about sadness and anger. When her mother went with her to the sessions, she also avoided talking to her. During the multidisciplinary staff meetings, it was decided that the mother should take part in the music therapy sessions. A hammock and Ayala's favorite games from home were brought to the therapy room. The goal was to recreate the same atmosphere as her home and transform the therapy room into a safe and enabling place that would serve as a transitional space between her home and the hospital. As early as the third session, Ayala began talking to her mother in the room and in the hall. Her mother told the music therapist which songs she listened to at home, and those songs were made part of the therapeutic process. Ayala grew up in a very warm and happy home and the selection of songs was upbeat and playful in contrast to her original choice of songs. In this way, the songs served as a bridge to creating a transitional space between her home and the hospital. Progressively, Ayala began speaking to the music therapist and later to the rest of the staff. She would only whisper with some of them, but with others she spoke loudly and confidently. Integrating her mother into the therapeutic process impacted therapy significantly.

A Space for Establishing Connections

The students' physical limitations restrict their range of movement and force them to remain confined to indoor spaces at home and in the hospital space. Most students commute daily from their homes to the hospital and back in a special shuttle, and routinely encounter the same people in similar contexts. The arts and animal-assisted therapy at Alyn Hospital provide an opportunity to create interesting and new connections between these patients and their social and natural surroundings which would otherwise be inaccessible.

The connection between the hospital staff and the students. Certain staff members at Alyn Hospital do not have direct contact with hospitalized patients. These include the management and the computing, finance, maintenance and cleaning staff. As part of an entrepreneurial course the staff attended, non-medical hospital staff members expressed the desire to become better acquainted with the patients. As a follow-up to this course, Yael Kalfus, the arts therapist, initiated an "Open Studio" project which included collaborative creative sessions between staff members who do not have contact with the patients and students from the school and rehabilitation classes. The goal was to reinforce the relationship between patients and staff members from the non-medical sectors. Yael conducted preparatory meetings with the staff where she provided background and explanations about the disabilities patients in general must cope with. Subsequently, 3 one hour meetings between the staff and the students were held in the art therapy room. The first session was an introductory encounter where the staff introduced themselves and described their departments and their respective roles. The students stated their names and ages. Then, Yael read the book "This is Not a Box" (Fortis, 2010), which is about a child who has a box, and in his imagination transforms it into different things. The adults and students split into mixed groups, where each group was given a cardboard box. Three sessions were devoted to designing and making artworks together from this material. Thereafter the students visited the staff members in their departments. At the conclusion of the sessions, an exhibition was held where all the artworks were displayed.

This project created a new, vital connection between the non-medical hospital staff and the students. The staff members were pleasantly surprised by the students' original ideas and discovered their own hidden talents during the process. However, these unconventional sessions were also a cause for concern that elicited reservations and embarrassment for both the adults and the students. Nevertheless, the staff members considered that these sessions strengthened their connection and gave new meaning to their work at the hospital, and the students were pleased to have had the opportunity to demonstrate their abilities, and to expand their social circle to adults and children from different wards in the hospital.

A connection between interior and exterior spaces. The variety of people at Alyn Hospital is striking. Beyond their many differences, the students share something in common in that they are all faced with severe health problems, deal with mobility issues and experience relative isolation from the outside world. Sessions with animals provide an opportunity for them to experience the natural world and let components of the outside world into the classrooms. The art, the music and experiencing animals and nature facilitate the creation of a space for dialogue between students and adults from different cultures.

Haggai Yoel, the animal-assisted therapist recalls:

> In my sessions with the students, we don't only work with the animals in the petting zoo, but also relate to the entire natural world. During one of the sessions when I was sitting with the students in the petting zoo, a flying ant flew towards us. They were not familiar with this species and I explained the nuptial flight phenomenon. The topic was later addressed in all the classes during the fall season. We became familiar with the world of ants, their different roles in the nest, and also drew the ants' routes as they flew. Yael, the art therapist, was also involved and worked with the students using toilet paper rolls to create ants and designate them according to their roles in the nest.

Learning about medicinal plants is another way to integrate the natural world into the classrooms. Herbal species from the Judean Mountains such as Salvia fruticose (sage), Micromeria fruticose (white leaved savory) and za'atar (a condiment) were brought into the classroom. The students studied the appearance of the plants, their smell and their taste, a learning experience that involved all the senses. In the Arabic-speaking classes, the students learned the names in Arabic. In the rehabilitation class, where some parents stay with their children, an encounter for parents and children of different cultures was set up. They discovered what the different cultures had in common by learning about the plants that grow near their homes. The direct encounter with nature and the world of senses helped to break down barriers, strengthen their connection to wildlife and the Earth and emphasize what they have in common.

The students also learned about the blossoming of various wildflowers. In the transition between fall and winter, the students were taught about Colchicum (autumn crocus), Crocus and Sternbergia (fall daffodil). They learned that the flowers can teach them about the seasons of the year, that the transition between seasons is gradual and the result is a very colorful and remarkable scene. Another opportunity to incorporate nature into the classrooms was presented when the students learned about spring blossoms. Most of them cannot go outside, so they enjoyed the spring flowers that Haggai collected for them in the field. After this experiential-sensory session, the students worked in small groups with Yael and drew the blooming fields of flowers.

Their encounter with the natural world allowed them to become exposed to the traditions, customs and folklore of different nations. When different wildflowers were brought to the classroom, their names were also presented in Arabic. When the students were studying about Colchicum, one of the Arab assistants mentioned that the name in Arabic means "the witch's lamp." The origin of the name is part of the folklore from her village. Later, the story was also told in the Hebrew classes and thus created an intercultural bridge connecting the students and staff from different backgrounds.

National holidays and memorial days are a sensitive and complex issue at the school where Jews and Arabs study together and raises questions and controversy over the different identities and loyalties of both students and staff. The therapy team, together with the educational staff, work to plan activities on these occasions that emphasize their shared values to avoid tensions between individuals of different identities, and simultaneously contribute towards enhancing the rich diversity at the hospital. For instance, before Jerusalem Day (an Israeli national holiday commemorating the reunification of Jerusalem) the arts therapist and the teachers decided to make models of different neighborhoods of the city with the students. Over the course of several weeks, each class worked in art therapy group sessions on the subject of "home." They used cardboard boxes and designed a home with different types of entrances and colors made from a range of art and recycling materials. At the same time, they also learned about the city and its neighborhoods with the teachers and planned the neighborhood that they wanted to build together. On Jerusalem Day, the classes assembled in the school auditorium, each seated around a large table, and laid out their own new neighborhood, thus building the character and spirit of the city.

Room for Initiative

The staff makes a consistent effort to find solutions to help overcome the students' physical limitations to facilitate direct contact with animals and art that can promote their therapeutic goals.

Accessibility. Many students enjoy seeing the animals at the petting zoo and ask to be moved closer to see them and touch them. For students in wheelchairs, it is much easier to bring the animals to them, but this does not allow them to see the animals in their natural environments, and thus restricts their encounter. Haggai Yoel, the animal-assisted therapist, initiated a different type of session in which the students interact with the animals at their level, despite the challenge of taking them out of their wheelchairs with their respiratory support systems. The rabbit hutches and guinea pig pens in the petting zoo are padded with mattresses, so the students can sit or lie and feed the animals vegetables. The animals come up to eat, and the students can watch them in their natural environment. The students' reactions to this first encounter were very touching. Those who were slightly worried about being too close to the animals were willing to give it a chance. They overcame their reservations and had a positive experience. One of the girls who reportedly refused to cooperate in physical and occupational therapy made an effort to sit up to feed the guinea pigs. She subsequently showed more willingness to cooperate during other paramedical treatments. The students realized that the animals were creatures of freedom and choice, thereby expanding their understanding of their encounter with them. They could sit near them while the animals moved around them or moved away. This experience was also processed in later conversations on choices and respecting animals as living creatures.

Using technology. In the advanced class, there are five students between the ages of nine and 21 with severe mobility disabilities. Three use alternate means of communication. Each student has a laptop connected to the wheelchair with a custom-designed switch to activate it: one student operates the computer with his eyes using a focal system, another uses his finger and the third uses her shoulder and fingers. Due to their physical limitations, the focus of the art therapy sessions is to facilitate choice. They choose what materials to work with and give the assistants precise instructions. In this class, Yael Kalfus initiated a session of creative animation work on the computer using the animation technique "stop motion" where the illusion of motion is created from a sequence of still shots of objects in slightly different positions in every image. The students' small movements steered the movement of the images in the animated film, reinforcing the experience of visibility, presence and accomplishment. The hospital agreed to purchase this software. Yael presented a stop-motion animation video to the students and explained the principles of animation. The occupational therapist adapted a photography switch for each student in the class. The students wrote personal stories on their computers, created a set of characters and started filming. The work was challenging: some of the students immediately understood the technique, while others found it difficult to comprehend. The work required a great deal of time and effort, but eventually a collaborative film was created by all the students in the class.

Breaking the taboo of talking about death. At Alyn Hospital, there are students with severe chronic illnesses, some of whom have life-threatening conditions. The students are often forced to cope with the sudden death of a classmate. The educational staff who also deal with hardships in these situations found it difficult to mediate these sensitive issues to the students and chose to shelter them from the difficult news by avoiding the subject of death. As a result, there was no mourning and separation process.

In view of this situation, the team of arts and animal-assisted therapists undertook to break the taboo and addressed the issue using the Kübler-Ross (1995) open and accepting approach that transcends the fear of death and directly addresses it. This approach highlights the power of symbolic language as a universal, spontaneous and honest means of communication, and as a way to process the confrontation with death. The team of therapists initiated a series of sessions, initially with the educational staff and the assistants. The participants were encouraged to express the subject of death through art and music. The participants shared personal experiences about death, including coping with the loss of students. They had the opportunity to experience an emotional outlet, feel supported and offer support to others. However, some expressed difficulties with the subject and struggled to address it directly. This led to the decision that the emotional processing of grief and separation would be mediated in the classrooms by the arts therapies team. When a student passes away, a conversation is held in the classroom about him or her, a picture is hung on the wall and an allocated space is created where students can express their feelings directly. Classmates can create a farewell drawing for the deceased and can give it to the family in mourning. During the discussions in the classrooms, the students' direct and honest reactions were often surprising. In one conversation, a student asked where her deceased classmate had gone, and the arts therapist turned the question back to the student: "Where do you think he is?" The student replied: "He is playing in heaven with my brother who died." The hospital management subsequently decided to create a permanent framework for staff members to process issues of loss and grief through a "Mourning and Living" forum in the hospital. The forum meets once a month throughout the year and all staff members from the health, education and rehabilitation professions are invited to attend. The forum is facilitated by the school psychologist and consists of lectures about palliative medicine and the processing of staff members' inevitable encounter with death.

Summary and Conclusions

The school at Alyn Hospital is a special treatment center where students from various sectors of society with severe physical disabilities are united by a common theme: the desire and effort to recover and rehabilitate. The school staff promotes a holistic approach that strives to address the needs of each patient's body, mind and spirit. The school provides unusual opportunities to work with an integrated team of medical, rehabilitative, educational and arts and animal-assisted therapists. The arts therapists' work focuses on creating partnerships and connections between professionals from different fields to promote the welfare of each student. The team of therapists at Alyn Hospital adheres to a working model that views the complexities and diversities inherent to the system as a creative challenge and an opportunity for initiative and growth. The working model is both expressive and supportive and emphasizes adaptation and rehabilitation. The art, music and animal-assisted therapies are crucial outlets for expression at Alyn Hospital. They serve as a conduit for hope, and integrate internal and external content, at different levels of functioning, for different languages and cultures, sickness and health.

The model also embeds the creativity and flexibility required of arts and animal-assisted therapists who work in an unconventional setting and proves that it is possible to create and maintain a therapeutic space in very challenging conditions. The experience at Alyn suggests that communication and collaboration between professionals in a multidisciplinary team contributes towards the shared goal of a comprehensive and inclusive understanding of each student's needs and the promotion of well-being. This model may thus be appropriate for schools in pediatric wards and in frameworks for students with severe disabilities who are treated by multidisciplinary staff.

References

Anzieu, D. (2016). *The skin-ego*. London: Karnac.

Bion, W.R. (2004). *Learning from experience*. New York: Jason Aronson.

Bowlby, J. (1990). *A secure base: parent-child attachment and healthy human development*. Michigan University: Basic Books.

Browne, A. (2006). *Silly Billy*. London: Walker Books.

Curry, N.A., & Kasser, T. (2005). Can coloring mandalas reduce anxiety? *Art Therapy*, *22*(2), 81–85.

Donaldson, J., & Scheffler, A. (2016). *Room on the broom*. United Kingdom: Pan Macmillan.

Favara-Scacco, C., Smirne, G., Schiliro, G., & Di Cataldo, A. (2001). Art therapy as support for children with leukemia during painful procedures. *Medical and Pediatric Oncology*, *36*(4), 474–480.

Fortis, A. (2010). *It's not a box*. Tel Aviv: Yedioth Ahronoth-Hemed. (in Hebrew).

Geva, N. (2009). I do not want. In *I have it all: Original songs and sounds of the big world (CD)*. Tel Aviv: Acum. (in Hebrew).

Hazut, T, & Segev-Shoham, A. (2002). The power of creativity in the works of hope and the experience of attachment between therapist and patient In A. Pinchover (Ed.), *The black colors died and the happy colors won - cancer drawings by children* (pp. 202–211). Tel Aviv: Hakibbutz Hameuchad (in Hebrew).

Kübler-Ross, E. (1995). *Death is of vital importance*. New York: Station Hill Press.

Malchiodi, C.A. (1999). *Medical art therapy with children*. London: Jessica Kingsley Publishers.

Nainis, N., Paice, J.A., Ratner, J., Wirth, J.H., Lai, J., & Shott, S. (2006). Relieving symptoms in cancer: innovative use of art therapy. *Journal of Pain and Symptom Management*, *31*(2), 162–169.

Saltzberg, B. (2010). *Beautiful oops*. New work: Workman Publishers.

Winnicott, D.W. (1971). *Playing and reality*. Middlesex: Penguin.

5 "We Have Created You Peoples and Tribes That You May Know One Another" (Surat Al Hujurat, Quran)

Multicultural Aspects of Arts Therapies in the Educational System

Yael Bruno and Zakiah Massarwa

Introduction

The multicultural aspects of psychotherapy have attracted increased attention in the last two decades, motivated in part by rising immigration from African, Middle Eastern, Asian and South American countries to Europe and North America. The causes of immigration are diverse and include factors that drive emigrants out of their homelands, as well as incentives that draw them towards their destinations. For instance, wars leave countless traumatized victims in their wake. Ethnic and political tensions as well as climate change affect the viability of eking out a living in the country of origin. People can easily access the internet to learn about distant societies and cultures, and strive to immigrate there. As legal and illegal immigration continues to expand, scholars have highlighted the importance of attending to cultural diversity (Smooha, 2018). In most Western countries, both government bodies and lay organizations provide resources to support the integration of immigrants and refugees from diverse cultural, religious and lifestyle backgrounds, some of whom have lived through harrowing experiences. Their children are integrated into the educational systems, which presents unique challenges that require both thought and action.

Arts therapists working within the education system are often called upon to support the emotional, interpersonal and physiological needs of these children. Complex multicultural encounters arise in situations where therapists from a Western individualistic background engage in a client-therapist relationship with school children from a collectivistic traditional society. The context of therapy within the Arab society of Israel was chosen here to illustrate the nature of this complex endeavor and its importance in arts therapy.

Theoretical Background

Cultural Identity and Intercultural Encounters

Throughout the previous century and even more so in the last two decades, numerous minority groups have begun to demand their rightful place in cultural, religious, economic and political discourse. In the United States, since the 1960s, what initially began as a movement in the African-American community has spread to other ethnic and religious minority groups (Hispanic-, Asian- and Native-Americans, to name a few). Even those who define themselves as socially excluded minorities within mainstream society, such as women, people with disabilities and people with various sexual orientations and identities, now insist on defining themselves as belonging to a distinct culture that differs from mainstream culture. This struggle is directed towards achieving greater social justice, legal egalitarianism and a proper share of the economic resources. Understandably, such struggles can be viewed as a threat to the hegemonic majority (Talwar, 2015).

These social processes resonate with the growing awareness of the multicultural aspects of psychotherapy, which occur whenever the therapist and the client belong to different cultural, social, familial or even gender backgrounds. Nowadays, many maintain that any encounter between two individuals is inevitably an intercultural one, where each party brings along his or her own cultural circles. Intercultural discourse simply sheds light on existing disparities (McNiff & Barlow, 2009; Moodley & Walcott, 2010).

Across different modes of therapy, these developments have prompted calls to better define the situation where two individuals who do not belong to the same culture, or where one or both do not belong to the hegemonic culture, can still function as a psychotherapeutic dyad. Can they understand each other's experiences, or even use the same language? Are therapists' worldview an obstacle to acknowledging the life experiences of their clients? For example, can there be a therapeutic relationship between a Caucasian therapist and an African-American client whose ancestors were slaves (Landy, 2008)? What would happen if hostility, including severe violent acts, were known to have taken place between the therapist's and the client's cultural groups in the past or the present? The therapeutic dynamic is especially susceptible to a variety of projections affecting both transference and countertransference, and may delay or completely block the therapeutic process.

Initially, the working assumption was that a therapist who was aware of intercultural differences could ignore them and strive to achieve a type of therapeutic "color blindness" (McNiff & Barlow, 2009). Shaun McNiff, one of the pioneering art therapists to study interculturalism in therapy, concurred with Freud that "basic psychic processes are universally present in all human experience and there is a fundamental 'psychic unity' to behavior in the present and past" (p. 101). This perspective assumes that people who originate from different cultures but want to assimilate into Western countries should gradually adapt and accept prevalent *Western* values and lifestyles (Sue & Sue, 1999; Talwar, Iyer, & Doby-Copeland, 2004). This notion of a unified consciousness underlying psychological processes and structures is often associated with Western hegemony. In the last two decades many activists and researchers have rejected this position as a form of *ethnocentric monoculturalism*.

More recently, there has been greater acknowledgment of the ways in which cultural differences can affect psychological assessment and evaluation, mental diagnoses and therapeutic goals. These biases can affect the therapist's ability to feel empathy towards the client, the client's confidence in being understood by the therapist and achieving full confidence (Potash et al., 2015). According to Talwar, Iver and Doby-Copeland (2004), it is precisely the awareness of intercultural disparities, alongside the therapist's own self-awareness, that constitutes the key to bridging this chasm: "A general myopia and color blindness among the dominant group impede the development of cultural competence… . Self-recognition and awareness of each art therapist and human being is the key to becoming an effective clinician" (p. 46). Based on the clinical experiences of therapists who have worked with disadvantaged minorities and advocacy on the part of the few African-American members of the American Art Therapy Association, the latter updated its ethics code in 2011 to include a detailed section discussing the ethical aspects of intercultural art therapy (AATA, 2013).

The psychotherapy literature implements various terms for the therapeutic relationship between therapist and client, each of which identifies with a different ethnic or cultural society. According to Zoabi and Savaya (2015), this terminology is directly influenced by the *zeitgeist* – the political correctness of the time. During the 1970s and 1980s, the therapist tended to belong to the majority culture and the client belonged to a minority group. Consequently, the terms *dual perspective* and *ethnic sensitivity* were used to denote the therapist's awareness and acknowledgment of sociocultural aspects and their meaning in the client's life. In the 1990s, the term *culturally sensitive* was coined in an attempt to integrate universal with culturally dependent aspects. Recently the term *culturally proficient* has been suggested. Here, therapists are expected to develop not only knowledge about their clients' cultures, but also skills that incorporate therapeutic practices derived from the clients' inner world, integrated with academic and professional practices. Furthermore, therapists must develop self-awareness of their own values and beliefs and their cultural heritage through a dialogue with those of their clients. In this chapter we utilize the term *cross-cultural* to portray the therapeutic relationships between individuals who belong to cultures embroiled in a complex relationship that includes conflicts and hostilities in the past and present.

Intercultural Therapy as an Inter-Paradigm Therapy

The issue of multiculturalism is germane even when both therapist and client identify with the same social group. Dwairy (2015) describes two social paradigms to categorize societies regardless of their technological or modern attributes: a democratic-liberal-Western paradigm vs. a traditional-collectivistic one. A traditional society regards the needs of the individuals as subordinate to the greater good of the collective, whether this is the family, clan, ethnic group or nation. Therefore, when in psychological crisis, the individual should seek help from a traditional healer or religious authority who will guide this person towards resuming socially accepted behavior. By contrast, Western psychotherapy encourages clients to aim for greater autonomy, self-awareness and realization of their potential. Dwairy maintains that the attempt to treat clients within a collectivistic society with interventions derived from a Western perspective creates substantial difficulties. Despite benevolent intentions on the part of therapists, they may not be in a position to help clients who desire or can even partake of such therapy. The client's cultural heritage is not always wholly obvious to the therapist. At times only nuances rooted in a specific culture can mobilize the client to fully engage in psychological processes of change. There is evidently a need for a dialogue of a different kind between therapist and client within this complex process, and doubly so when therapy occurs within the educational system where the therapist is perceived by both students and parents as an authority figure and a member of the educational system.

Description of the Working Model and Clinical Examples

This section delves into the specific issue of art therapy in Israeli public education, specifically when directed towards its Arab minority groups. The Special Education Law of 1988 mandated access to art therapies in the school system. Within the last 20 years, art therapy has become the psychotherapy of choice, and is available to almost any student aged 3–18 in need. Providing this service to Arabic-speaking children entailed a vast training process of young arts therapists from the Arab minority, a vocation previously unheard of in this sector. The brief description below presents the social background and current situation of the Arab minority in the State of Israel, as it impacts arts therapies in the school system.

The Sociopolitical Background in the State of Israel

The demographical situation in the State of Israel is complex in that it includes individuals from different religious and ethnic groups that speak different languages. This has historical roots that continue to shape the State of Israel to this day, as well as the deep-seated conflicts within its population. The crux of the conflict is tied to the incompatible perspective of the disparate Jewish and Arab peoples regarding rights to the land. This complex situation has created layered identities for Arabic-speaking Israeli citizens: apart from their individual and gendered identities, they also have an Arabic cultural identity, a specific ethnic identity (e.g., Bedouin), a religious identity (e.g., Muslim, Christian, Druze) and a Palestinian national identity. We use the term "Israeli Palestinian/Arab (IPA)" because it best describes the wide range of self-definitions with conflicting political and national interpretations referring to Arabic-speaking Israeli citizens, who are mostly identified with the Palestinian nation while valuing their Israeli citizenship.

Arab Society in Israel at Present

According to the Central Bureau of Statistics (2018), the Arab society in Israel is an ethnic minority numbering approximately 1,838,200 people, who comprise around 20.9% of Israel's demographics. It is composed of three main religious groups: Muslims (83.8%), Christians (8.4%) and Druze (8.2%). Arabs have a lower socioeconomic status than their Jewish counterparts: lower quality education (Abu-saad, 2004), higher unemployment rates or employment in unskilled or low-skilled professions, a low-income level (about 34% below the national average) and high poverty rates (54% compared to 19% of all families in Israel) (Institution for Social Security, 2015). There are also huge gaps in living conditions between the groups, as Arab neighborhoods are characterized by high poverty, infrastructure and neighborhood problems, including crime, violence and road safety issues (Daoud, Sergienko, O'Campo, & Shoham-Vardi, 2017).

Arab society is traditional at its core, and incorporates several characteristics of a collectivistic culture. It emphasizes values which serve the group over the individual, such as strong familial ties, harmonic bonds and interdependence (Dwairy, 1998; Dwairy, 2002). It can also be described as patriarchal, patrilineal and hierarchical. Arab society stresses the importance of conformism and mutual respect as the essential moral values of human relations, as well as harmony with one's surroundings. Therefore, it is considered preferable to solve problems within the family unit rather than utilize the services provided by the state. Al-Haj (1989) considers the Arab minority in Israel to be a society in transition, caught between Eastern and Western cultures due to the process of Westernization within Israel. This cultural clash between Western culture and traditional Arab culture has shaped a plethora of developments that are closely related to educational issues, including those related to arts therapy.

Arts Therapy Enters the Arab Educational System in Israel

The passing of the Special Education Act (SEA) in 1988 regulated the rights of students with special needs. Between 1996 to1998, an operative plan for the implementation of this law was drawn up. These included establishing therapeutic centers for special education in urban centers and in key locations within rural areas. These centers were entrusted with operating paramedical services such as physical therapy, occupational therapy, speech therapy, as well as arts therapies. These services were given within the centers, and gradually reached out to special education kindergartens and schools. In the State of Israel, there are two distinct and separate educational systems, one for Jewish students and one for Arabs. Given the national nature of the new budget, these centers were launched in nearly equal quantities and quality throughout the country and required urgent staffing. Consequently, children from Arab society were suddenly given an opportunity to benefit from therapies and services which were unavailable before.

Phase 1: Implementing the SEA – Jewish Therapists Working in Arab Society (1998–2008)

Working Conditions – the Setting. As appeared in the previous paragraph, therapeutic support centers were established in Arab towns and rural areas, and IPA directors were appointed to oversee them. For political, cultural and social reasons, the physical infrastructure of the educational institutes in Arab settlements is quite challenging in comparison to their Jewish counterparts (Al-Haj, 1995). This directly affects arts therapy in that the school structures are older and poorly maintained, there are fewer available therapy rooms and there is meager funding for equipment and materials (Snir et al., 2018). Therapists who began working in Arab schools thus sought out their own creative solutions; group therapy took place in the special education classrooms, less than adequate rooms (such as those used by the school nurse or counselor, or even as storerooms) were refitted to be dual-purpose, and the therapists used different rooms throughout the workweek. Therapists who lasted in a given institution managed through constant negotiations with the principal to find solutions that allowed therapy to take place.

The therapists. Initially, the few IPA arts therapists in Israel were those certified abroad, all of whom were men. Women were prohibited from such qualifications due to the cultural-social ban on unaccompanied female travel (Abu Baker, 2008). Only a handful of female Arab students were able to study in arts therapy training institutions in Israel. Therefore, Jewish therapists were hired to work in Arab schools, usually without knowing any Arabic and without preparation or designated training about Arab society. Their personal experiences are easily comparable to those of Western therapists treating newly arrived immigrants and refugees (Quinlan, Schweitzer, Khawaja, & Griffin, 2015), or therapists who travel to treat children in war-torn, disaster-struck or Third World countries (Ahmed & Siddiqi, 2006; Behrens, 2019).

What sets Israeli-Jewish therapists apart is that they did not come for a limited period of time, and were not required to distance themselves from their families and country of origin. Furthermore, the cultural gap between them and their clients involved not only linguistic, religious and cultural issues but it also had a distinctly political tonality. The Jewish arts therapists who chose to work in Arab locations did so because it entailed supporting a disadvantaged minority, or out of political idealism. A similar choice was documented, for example, by Haen (2007) who described his work as a White American therapist treating African-American clients, and Sideris (2017) who discussed a case involving an Aboriginal Australian client. In these cases, the therapeutic relationships involved the encounter between distinct cultures with a conflictual historical and social background.

The arts therapists were often the only Jewish personnel within an all-Arab educational institute. They were unable to communicate with the students or their families in their mother tongue. Julia Kristeva (1991) poetically described a similar experience:

> not speaking one's mother tongue. Living with resonances and reasoning that are cut off from the body's nocturnal memory, from the bittersweet slumber of childhood. Bearing within oneself like a secret vault, or like a handicapped child – cherished and useless – that language of the past that withers without ever leaving you.
>
> (pp. 15–16)

Attempts were made to provide a translator for the sessions. This effort proved problematic in that it both violated confidentiality but also crimped the development of a therapist-client bond (Chilcote, 2007). Focusing on the arts as the central channel of communication has its own advantages over emphasizing speech (Robb, 2002). The therapists thus opted to rely primarily on arts, with minimal verbal conversation in Hebrew (a language their clients did not understand or preferred not to use). Another preferred option was to co-lead bilingual group therapy with a non-therapist member of the school staff, usually the special education primary teacher or the school counselor. This solution promoted modeling and mutual learning where both members became acquainted with the personal as well as organizational culture of his/her peer, thus enhancing the well-being of the student clients. Those Jewish therapists who chose to continue working within Arab society recognized the need to voluntarily invest in attaining at least a basic grasp of Arabic, as well as become acquainted with Arab culture both formally and informally through art, music, literature, cinema, etc.

Language barriers were not the only challenge of this cross-cultural encounter. A Jewish therapist who does not speak Arabic is often unaware of cultural nuances of the gendered and school hierarchy. Every interaction with school staff members has repercussions at the sociopolitical level since the therapist is often regarded as a representative of the ruling Jewish majority. The stereotypes and prejudices of the therapist, the clients and their families, and the educational staff pave the way for mutual projections. Srour (2015) discussed the feelings of distress, confusion, anger and helplessness of Jewish therapists during memorial days for Jewish casualties killed during wars with neighboring Arab countries and terror attacks involving Palestinians. During times of war or violent political incidents, the situation became more complex. For example, one Jewish art therapist described a meeting with an adolescent Muslim client who bluntly stated: "You are killing us!". When she replied with a question – "Did I do so myself?" – her client answered: "*You* didn't." This verbal exchange led to a conversation about the roots of her anger. In a wider context, Srour argued that this cultural transference-countertransference dynamic could serve as a catalyst for such major therapeutic issues as trust, ambivalence, anger and acceptance of disparate parts of the self.

The understanding of self-disclosure and the maintenance of a therapeutic setting are very different in Arab society as compared to Jewish society. The following Arab proverb expresses the key difference: "ان ضلت في القلب بتجرح وان طلعت لبرا بتفضح," that is: "if you keep it inside of you – it breaks your heart; if you let it out – it shames you" (Massarwa, 2016). The issue of revealing and concealing familial secrets takes on different meanings in Arab society (Dwairy & Van Sickle, 1996). The therapist's insistence on agreeing to a fixed timetable for meetings, or ensuring that therapy takes place in a closed, private room can elicit resistance on the part of the school staff (Snir et al., 2018). Therapists soon discovered that flexibility and a willingness to ask questions on any subject whatsoever of the staff, parents and colleagues helped solve most problems related to the workplace.

Specialized supervision. The Jewish therapists working in Arab locations felt the need for specialized supervision. According to Dwairy and Van Sickle (1996), culturally sensitive supervision helps therapists realize that therapy is not the place for criticism or for addressing the possible shortcomings of the client's culture. In 1998–1999, Tamar Hazut, one of the pioneers of arts therapy in Israel, launched a supervision group for arts therapists working in IPA society designed to enhance the cultural sensitivity of its participants (Roth-Yaniv, Mayan, & Hazut, 1999). The group discussed the research literature and invited Arab guest lecturers to speak. During a seminar on the Arab-Jewish encounter in psychotherapy, Shafik Masalha (in Vardimon, 2011) suggested that:

> Allowing different emotions engendered by the Jewish-Arab encounter to surface, even when they involve strong emotions such as fear, anger, and hatred, is the only viable approach for the creation of a safe space that may cease to be governed by these feelings, but will rather contain them.

Therapists began considering these interactions as an opportunity to open the political Pandora's Box and evolve beyond projections and maxims into a personal introspection on their emotions. One such example was provided by a Jewish therapist working in a Druze high school on the annual Memorial Day for the Fallen of the Israeli Defense Forces, which takes place on the eve of Independence Day. Druze men enlist in the Israeli army, and thus Memorial Day is celebrated in school. In her words:

> I entered the teachers' lounge on Memorial Day. A Muslim teacher I work with, sat by herself, apart from the others, and did not take part in the military ceremony that was being held at the school. I listened to her as she told me about how her parents had been driven into exile during the *Nakbah.*
>
> {War of 1948 – *catastrophe* as referred to by the Palestinians}

Phase 2: "First Generation"- pioneer IPA Arts Therapists

Many Jewish therapists felt that learning Arabic and acquiring some familiarity with the culture was a rudimentary requirement for successful therapy. They thus considered that they were simply working temporarily until enough IPA arts therapists could be qualified, and could work as therapists and supervisors within their own culture. The next section describes the efforts made towards achieving this complex endeavor, which can be conceptualized as the *birth pangs* of IPA arts therapy.

Recruitment and training of students from Arab society. The demands of the training procedure in arts therapy training institutes were considered challenging by IPA arts therapy students, and recruiting efforts were often slow or unsuccessful. Awais and Yali (2013) described efforts to recruit African-American candidate therapists among graduates of both public and African-American colleges in the US. They emphasized that "diversity in the classroom can offer novel perspectives on theory, practice and research. Greater diversity of art therapists would allow clients the opportunity to choose a practitioner who identifies as a member of a racial or ethnic minority" (p. 130).

Word of the new profession circulated gradually among IPA students in similar professions such as psychology, social work and education, encouraging them to seek qualification in arts therapy. The first women to join this profession saw themselves and were seen by their Jewish milieu as "pioneers, first and foremost for their very choice to study a profession which is little known in general and particularly unfamiliar in their society" (Angel, 2014, p. 9). These women acted as role models for other women on school staffs, the families of their clients and in their communities and were considered catalysts of deep-seated changes in society.

Hurdles facing IPA women interested in studying arts therapies. The experience of an isolated female IPA arts therapy student studying in a Jewish university or college, in a Jewish town far from her place of residence, is often that of singularity and alienation. Hebrew and English are the languages of study, which are second and third languages for her. Leaving the close-knit circle of family and hometown, at times with only limited support from family members who are unfamiliar with the vocation and its implications, often compel female students to make an immense personal, social and economic effort. Arar and Abu-Rabia-Queder emphasized that "cultural norms in developing countries assume that people should act in accordance with gender expectations...and women who attempt to achieve this type of role risk incurring cultural sanctions such as reduced chances for marriage" (2011, p. 416). A pioneering art therapist told us:

> My professional choice to study arts therapy came from a conscious inner place, it's a field that I myself am interested in, not something that societal pressures have pushed me into. It expresses the courage of an Arab woman of our day and age to say: this fits me and that doesn't fit me! It's a feminist revolt: breaking the hold of the collective when it comes to choosing my own career.

In Israel, the field of arts therapy, unlike teaching in primary and secondary education, requires both a BA and an MA. The implications for an IPA student are not only that the financial expenses are doubled, but also that she cannot fulfill her traditional role as housekeeper or support herself and her family during those years (Massarwa, 2016). The first students in this field experienced the encounter with Jewish society as complicated, often conflictual, but nurturing and empowering, an encounter that elicited a new awareness of her complex identity. The story of one of them emphasizes this complexity:

> I was the first Palestinian, the only one in my [art therapy] class. We were asked to select the artwork of a famous painter. We were given the task of analyzing that artwork from a psychological perspective and identifying possible pathological characteristics in the art. I chose a famous Palestinian artist and my teacher said she had never heard of him. I insisted on my choice of examining an artist from my own culture and society.

In the US, the high tuition to earn a degree in arts therapies is a major factor preventing students from minority cultures from choosing this career. In Israel, families of IPA students are deeply involved in the decisions regarding choice of career and financing tuition, even though the cost of a college education is subsidized by the government. Thus, the major factor preventing IPA students and their families from choosing to study arts therapies is the lack of acquaintance with the profession.

Publicizing the new profession and recruiting IPA students. Several attempts have been made to address these issues. When starting in a new institution, the arts therapists were asked to provide several *arts therapy workshops* in each class in their school. This enabled the teachers and the principals to get a sense of the therapeutic value of arts therapy for their students. In addition, the arts therapists initiated *continuing education (CE) programs* for school counselors, regular and special education school and kindergarten teachers focusing on the emotional needs of children and the role of arts therapy in alleviating them.

"Preparatory year" programs for arts therapies

In conversations with practicum supervisors, several concerns were raised regarding the integration of IPA students in arts therapy programs. Several disparities between IPA students and Jewish students were mentioned: IPA students tended to be unfamiliar with psychology as a discipline, and were much less experienced and knowledgeable in the arts. Jewish students arrived with some basic knowledge of the arts learned in the Jewish educational system or through informal study of the arts. Arts courses both formal and informal are generally inaccessible in Arab society. Likewise, there is a pronounced discrepancy between the liberal Western perspective and the traditional Arab view of art. In Western perspectives, art is considered as an outlet for emotional and individualized expression. By contrast, art in traditional Arab society is a collective experience that evokes traditional customs (e.g., Dabke dance as opposed to modern dance; calligraphy and arabesque vs. modern art, etc.). Gender may play a crucial role in stage arts such as drama and singing: a woman's choice to participate in public performances might be perceived as indecent.

The teachers in arts therapy training programs are mainly acculturated members of Western as well as Jewish society (considered to be midway between individualistic and collectivistic society) and refer predominantly to Western or Jewish art, music, theater and dance. Non-Western hegemonic artists receive little or no attention. Hence, an arts therapy student who belongs to a minority group may suffer from twofold exclusion: both her own, and that of the culture she was raised in. Angel (2014), a faculty member in a bibliotherapy program, described the alienation felt by IPA students since only Hebrew texts from Jewish culture were studied in class. She invited them to bring texts from their own culture, read them aloud in Arabic (a language usually marginalized in public) and translate them to their peers. This elicited a wide range of emotional responses, including strong political ones.

The kind of therapy taught in the practicum is derived from the liberal Western paradigm. The primary goal of Western psychotherapy itself – that of empowerment through personal emotional expression – may be perceived as menacing, unacceptable and even dangerous when viewed from a traditional Arab perspective. Most Jewish students have greater familiarity with the practice of Western therapy, and some have undergone either psychotherapy or arts therapy as a client. According to Al-Krenawi and Graham (2011):

> Arab peoples in Israel may consider mental health systems as outside their cultures and having limited cultural fit (...) A number of factors may inhibit students' access to psychological care including fear of emotions, perception of stigma, fear of treatment, or reluctance to self-disclose.
>
> (pp. 164, 158)

Furthermore, the kind of psychotherapy available to students of low socio-economical standing is provided by the public healthcare system, which is predominantly staffed by Jewish therapists. Engaging in this type of psychotherapy can have significant political ramifications since it is often perceived as reaffirming the societal power imbalance and thus has a clear colonialist connotation.

The pursuit of arts therapy cannot avoid dealing with manifestations of societal and political values. The IPA arts therapy student is faced with a dilemma: can she freely express herself and risk experiencing the heavy cost of divulging her political opinions in class, or should she block her personal outlook to better fit her Jewish surroundings (Angel, 2014). Masalha (in Vardimon, 2011) describes a situation where the collective Arab unconscious and the collective Jewish unconscious clashed in the context of a psychology practicum:

> In a situation of conflict like the one Israel is embroiled in, the integrative and therapeutic goal may face numerous obstacles, including stereotypical and prejudiced beliefs of both therapists and clients, a predilection for projecting a view of evil as an outer force and good as an inner force, and by contrast the dissolution of diversity, which aims to lower anxiety levels by denying differences and otherness, and viewing the reality of what takes place in the room as isolated from what happens on the outside.

To counteract these disparities, the heads of the arts therapy training program at the University of Haifa decided to design a cost-free preparatory year in the domains of psychology and the arts. This program was addressed to mental health professionals (school counselors, psychologists and special education teachers) from Arab society interested in arts therapies degrees and careers. It was tailored to bridge the intercultural gap and the lack of previous opportunities in Arab society, and enable participants to prepare for the admission requirements.

Introducing an art therapy program designed for IPA therapists. In the mid-20th century, minority-serving institutions were established in the US. These colleges were designed specifically for students from ethnic minorities or members of the deaf and hard-of-hearing community. A similar program for IPA students was established in Maghar (a small town in northern Israel) in 2005, as an extension of Tel-Hai College. The program, led by Arab and Jewish faculty, operated for six academic years with approximately 90 graduating therapists, mostly IPAs. The graduates described their experiences as follows:

> "I would like every Arab woman to undergo the change I went through"
> "I learned to speak out my dreams, say what I want"
> "[being] traditional and religious, it is not right to dance and move freely"
> "[I] recalled my family's objection to my studies. Recalled all the people who told me: no, you are wasting time, you are doing nonsense, you are wrong, you are losing your children, you are mistaken."
> (Dror-Hadar, 2015, pp. 161–174)

The termination of this program raised many questions concerning the pros and cons of having an academic institute aimed specifically at Arab society. A discussion concerning the effectiveness and ethics of separate higher education was also addressed by the United States Commission on Civil Rights (2010), which focused on the 105 Historically Black Colleges and Universities (HBCUs). The findings showed clear advantages of studies in a separate setting for members of a social minority. Despite the disparity in level of education attained in the public high-school educational system (an estimated gap of up to four school years), students were able to enrol in scientific courses of study and achieved higher scores and more advanced degrees than those of their counterparts in predominantly White institutes. An accommodating environment, closer ties with their professors and a lack of prejudice and its stressors were all mentioned as explanations for their accomplishments. However, there are several drawbacks to separate programs: many students experienced difficulties when enrolling in advanced courses or entering the labor market, primarily because the quality of lecturers and academic demands in the separate institution are both lower than other academic institutes, as are the investments in infrastructure. The students felt inadequately equipped to handle what was "out there," and attested to difficulties in relationships with both other minorities and the hegemonic majority. The Supreme Court of the United States went so far as to raise the question of whether racially separated education is appropriate or beneficial in our day and age.

IPA students in an arts therapies practicum. During their courses, arts therapy IPA students took part in field work, mostly within Jewish society. The future IPA therapist encountered the inherent challenges of treating clients in Hebrew and within an Israeli-Jewish-dominant environment, which created a reversal of roles: the art therapy student belonging to the minority group served as the therapeutic authority with respect to clients belonging to the hegemonic group. Problems of compromised comprehension of the Hebrew language and knowledge of Jewish cultural codes led at times to complex and uncomfortable situations (Angel, 2014). Furthermore, a complication of a political nature occurred at times, whenever students or their families had difficulty accepting treatment from an Arab therapist. This could manifest as resistance to treatment, or even in open hostility. Srour (2015) warned of even greater dangers: "Unwanted parts of the therapists' ethnic identity (hatred, inferiority, discrimination) may also be dissociated and impact the therapy and the therapist's ability to feel empathy" (p. 409).

Supervision throughout the practicum was provided, for the most part, by Jewish supervisors who tended not to be trained in cross-cultural sensitivity. The difficulties facing an IPA student dealing with Jewish staff and clients was not always understood. The practicum supervision of student-therapists working in Arab society institutes was even more challenging. The supervisor often did not understand the intricacies, and forced the student-therapist to resolve conflicting social codes between the social norms prevalent in Arab society and those grounded in therapy. For example, when an IPA therapist brought up the case of a student suffering from abuse, the supervisor pressured her into immediate reporting in accordance with the mandatory report law. When she tried to uphold the law, the therapist encountered severe resistance from the school staff thus endangering the therapy. This dilemma will be further discussed below. IPA supervisees often adhere to what is acceptable behavior in traditional society; standing up to the supervisor or arguing with her are perceived as undermining her authority and thus improper conduct. At times, the supervisee opted not to mention emotional or political difficulties due to concerns about the supervisor's possible reaction, which could jeopardize her own professional prospects.

Phase 3: Passing the Torch – IPA Therapists Working in Their Own Society (2008–2020)

The next decade was characterized by greater outreach of arts therapies into the IPA community. As a result, a multitude of newly trained IPA arts therapists entered the public Arab education system. This section discusses the advantages as well as disadvantages of this process for therapists, clientele and supervision. New ethical dilemmas have arisen especially for the mandatory reporting of abuse.

The therapists. Gradually, IPA graduates of arts therapy programs filled the posts in the educational system, alongside veteran Jewish therapists, to cover most public Arab educational institutions. At present, over 200 IPA therapists are employed, allowing for gradual percolation and assimilation into other education institutions. Initially, schools were unable to identify which students would benefit from arts therapy. Terms such as *emotional* *or psychological difficulties* were perceived as highly intimidating, since they were seen as related to mental illness. Mental health diagnoses have societal stigma with long-term consequences for both students and their families (Snir et al., 2018). Arts therapy thus introduced an utterly novel paradigm: engaging in a creative activity accompanied by verbal processing that was considered to have a beneficial effect on the client's well-being while reducing the adverse symptoms evidenced in day-to-day school life.

Consequently, both the advantages and new difficulties associated with IPA therapists became apparent. In some areas, principals were unfamiliar with the new profession and prioritized "familiar" paramedical resources (e.g., occupational, speech or physical therapy) over arts therapies. Furthermore, it was widely expected that the few hours allocated to arts therapy would be equally apportioned to all educational frameworks, which would have resulted in a very small number of therapist hours for each school. Arts therapists were thus called upon to work in numerous educational settings and shuttle from one to another throughout the workday (Snir et al., 2018). This practice took its toll since it limited the therapist's availability to deal satisfactorily with obligations to school, parents and staff, such as interprofessional meetings and parental guidance.

The clientele – students and their families. Arab society is less affluent than Jewish society and subject to additional social and economic pressures. Many parents of students with special needs are unable to drive their children to a distant culturally foreign clinic, at the expense of work, family and economic obligations. Arts therapy in the school setting is readily available to all students, cost-free and flexible time-wise. Furthermore, there is less need for parental presence, making it better suited for this demographic.

Initially, arts therapy was viewed as alien and unknown. Parents opposed arts therapy, because they viewed it as a new form of psychological stigmatization by State authorities. Gradually, the provision of emotional therapy to students within the educational system proved beneficial. Contacts by parents with the school's paramedical staff proved discreet and confidential, and therapy has become more socially accepted. Clients' families react in different ways to the exposure of family secrets: some prefer to speak in their mother tongue with a therapist who understands the societal nuances, while others prefer divulging secrets to a "foreign" (i.e., Jewish) therapist, confident that their secrets will not be divulged (Snir et al., 2018).

Due to its indirect and metaphorical nature, arts therapy is often better suited to families of clients from Arab society. Direct divulging of negative emotions and unconscious content is considered improper. Through art making, these themes can be expressed, both symbolically and metaphorically (Dwairy, 2015). In IPA society, the term *psychologist* or *psychiatrist* often conveys a distinct stigma related to mental illness (Al-Krenawi & Graham, 2011). The therapist mediates the deeper significance of her vocation when dealing with parents by repeatedly explaining both the nature of her psychotherapeutic interventions and their limitations and boundaries.

Yet, outwardly, the parents can easily maintain a façade of absolute normalization, by claiming to relatives that their child is merely involved in an "art making." Most children react with exhilaration when presented with art materials and individualized attention (as noted above, Arab society is a collectivist environment with very few art classes in its schools). Consequently, arts therapy as a discipline has achieved substantial legitimation in the Arab educational system, and is on a par or often preferred to psychological therapy.

Ethical Considerations

FUNNELING BIAS: IPA ARTS THERAPISTS WORKING IN THEIR OWN SOCIETY

Given the growing numbers of IPA arts therapists, new decisions had to be made: should they return to work within Arab society or rather work alongside their Jewish counterparts in integrated public posts regardless of the cultural and language barriers? Within the medical system (including in-hospital educational staff), total equality and integration is the norm. IPA and Jewish medical personnel join hands in the treatment of IPA and Jewish patients. Unlike the medical system, education in Israel has been historically divided into separate Arab and Jewish systems along the language barrier. This has created a professional bias in that IPA therapists were encouraged by the education system to find work within the very same town and/or cultural-religious community whose language they speak and whose lifestyle they are familiar with. This bias was congruent with some therapists' own wishes to work in their hometown and thus avoid driving elsewhere (female driving after sundown is considered improper in certain communities). Such a professional choice was less challenging and reduced the need to cope with staff, clients and families belonging to a different ethnic, religious or national community. Promotion to the position of supervisor, coordinator or director was more readily available and involved less competition.

There are, however, significant drawbacks entailed in this choice; the therapist is exposed to external information regarding both her clients and their families which is passed around the town as gossip and can potentially impinge on the therapeutic process. Likewise, the families of her clients are also exposed to personal information about her and her family. This familiarity can affect their willingness to become her clients, and their attitude during treatment. Any prior acquaintance between therapist and client also challenges the former's capacity to maintain a neutral attitude as a therapist. Many Arab communities are characterized by close-knit extended families. Therapists employed in their hometown are likely to encounter distant relatives among school staff, social and other services who may press them to divulge confidential information. This situation further compromises their therapeutic freedom and presents a real threat to their professionalism. A multicultural team naturally enriches mutual learning within the team as well as benefits the clientele.

SOCIAL AND GENDER PRESSURES WITHIN ARAB SOCIETY

Ethical dilemmas tend to arise when principals utilized their power over young local therapists to manipulate professional decisions regarding allotment or continuation of therapy, referrals to another mode of therapy and other moves. Some school principals refused to allocate crucial resources such as a proper therapy room, equipment or materials. In one particular case, a principal forced a therapist to work as a teacher by threatening to fire her otherwise. The power differential between the principal and the Jewish therapists prevented such behavior.

INTER-ETHNIC THERAPY IN ARAB SOCIETY

Many Arab settlements are ethnically intermixed and include Muslim, Druze and Christian residents. An arts therapist working in her mother tongue but within a community other than her own can encounter inter-religious prejudices, or open hostility due to different political stances. For example, a Muslim arts therapist working in a Druze village (the latter serve in the Israeli Army, whereas Muslims do not), was met with violent and racist remarks concerning Arabs while conducting group therapy. The special education students were unaware of her identity, and freely expressed their aggressive fantasies as to their future army service. She deliberated in supervision when and how to disclose the fact that she is a Muslim, if at all. Another such case involved a Druze arts therapist working in a disadvantaged Muslim village with a rampant crime rate. When her car was vandalized, she felt unwelcome and directly targeted as a Druze in a Muslim environment.

MANDATORY REPORTING

Massarwa (2016) defined two conflicting principles in Arab society. People are warned against the social consequences of "speaking without thinking," which contrasts with the term *usturu* (استروا), which signifies the importance of keeping something protected and concealed to prevent the sharing of embarrassing or shaming information (p. 22). When an IPA therapist encounters a case of abuse, she sees the benefits for her client of confronting mistreatment and perhaps even stopping it. Yet mandatory reporting constitutes an impossible choice between adhering to her professional values as an arts therapist or adhering to her cultural responsibility to *usturu*, on the other. A Jewish therapist facing the same mandatory reporting requirement is considered by both family and school staff as a member of the hegemonic authorities and is thus expected to act according to the law. In both cases the report could result in harm to the client. The abused child is often blamed for the abuse itself, as well as for exposing a closely kept secret to the general public – a form of "ratting out." The reporting may put her in danger of revenge by family members or lead to suicide.

In addition, the report might be read by others involved in its filing (within the educational system, local government or social services) who has a familial relationship with the abuser's family or could be threatened. Interviews conducted by Massarwa found numerous cases where the secret and the identity of the reporter was leaked to the abuser's family, often leading to premature termination of therapy. Filing a mandatory report has personal repercussions for the IPA therapist as well; she might lose her job or suffer real threats to her life and property.

Abu Baker and Dwairy (2003) proposed an intervention program designed for IPA culture where prominent community and family figures, as well as local law and judicial enforcement, all ascertain the well-being of the victimized child, as well as that of his or her family. The abuser is punished or excommunicated and atones for his/her crimes in ways appropriate to his/her society.

Designing continuing education and culturally proficient supervision. Research has noted the lack of CE programs designed for the specific needs of arts therapists in Arab society (Snir et al., 2018). Issues such as difficulties stemming from intercultural differences within the diverse ethnic communities comprising the Arab society, the infiltration of societal and political stressors into therapy, the empowerment of therapists working in educational facilities lacking resources, acquaintance with Arab artists and expanding a customized artistic toolbox and so on are not addressed. In 2009, the needs of arts therapists employed in Arab society were first assessed. As a result, only two special CE courses for both Jewish and Arab arts therapists employed in Arab society were launched, led by Jewish instructors. In practice, there is further need for such courses.

Both the ethics committee and Arab society committee in the Israeli Association for Creative Arts Therapies (YAHAT) have been convened to deal with these ethical issues. In 2019, the Israeli Arts Therapy code of ethics was translated into Arabic and became the first and only such ethic code of arts therapy in the world. We believe that educating IPA therapists about these ethical issues, as well as continuous guidance through culturally sensitive supervision, can support the therapist by discussing these quandaries with staff and parents.

Recommendations

Several recommendations can be made.

1. **Enhancing the cultural-sensitivity of arts therapy faculty members and field supervisors.** IPA arts therapy students and therapists have often stated that training in cultural sensitivity would allow supervisors and teachers to discuss complex and volatile issues early on and support better familiarization of the students with the arts therapy profession. Introducing multicultural materials in the relevant field of

art (e.g., Arab music, Arab texts) could further alleviate the sense of alienation many IPA students feel (Angel, 2014). Jewish arts therapists who are veterans of the formative years of art therapy in Arab society have gradually become faculty members and supervisors. Their cultural proficiency, acquired in actual practice, was integrated into their teaching and supervision.

Initially, the supervisors appointed in each treatment center were all from Jewish society. Over the years, IPA therapists have been trained in supervision and are gradually replacing Jewish supervisors. To date, there are 15 IPA supervisors, nine of whom serve in the role of coordinators of arts therapy in their region. The local supervisor is knowledgeable about the functioning of Arab settlements, recognizes how and whom to approach when help is needed and has the necessary standing as an intermediary between therapists and principals (Snir et al., 2018). In recent years, the Ministry of Education has promoted training in the supervision of IPA arts therapists. Some of these supervisors continue their training in academic institutes in Israel and abroad, and have published papers and written their doctoral dissertations. We hope this development will eventually encourage acknowledged IPA scholars to join the arts therapy staff and engage in the training of future generations of IPA arts therapists.

2. **Promoting research and specific academic conferences.** The first conference aimed specifically at arts therapy in Arab society took place in Israel in 2016 under the sponsorship of the Israeli Association for Creative Arts Therapies (YAHAT). Since then, conferences have taken place biannually with a growing number of participants and presenters, primarily IPAs. In recent years, similar seminars have been held in arts therapy programs in their academic institutes as well. At the University of Haifa, field research on arts therapy in Arab society is continually being conducted (Snir et al., 2018). Awais and Yali (2013) pointed to the importance of encouraging research and active involvement in academic conferences to increase the percentage of minority students in arts therapy programs in the United States.

Limitations

The authors of this chapter are arts therapists who are deeply involved in the evolution of arts therapy in IPA society. Their attitude is therefore as insiders rather than a possibly more objective stance of external researchers. This chapter was written from an arts therapy point of view and does not include complementary perspectives such as those of school psychologists, representatives of the Division of Special Education, etc.

There is a question of generalizability: how relevant is the Israeli case to other countries with inter-ethnic or inter-religion social strife with a different historical background? Can the model described here be relevant to countries with altogether different public education systems? There is a lack of longitudinal research on the process of development described above. Such research would contribute to the literature and to practice and how it could be applied elsewhere.

Summary and Conclusions

This chapter illustrated the important role arts therapy can play within a multicultural society. In addition to ethnic and religious factors that characterize multicultural societies, Israeli society has unique political rifts threatening to tear apart its fragile social fabric. The chapter exemplifies how therapy provided by the government through public educational and healthcare systems can facilitate effective societal change. This type of public service enables better management of therapists' competence, supervision and continued professional training. The therapists feel supported and empowered when facing complex clientele.

Throughout the years, the impact of IPA therapists on their society has become that much more apparent. As pioneers within their society, they paved the way for emotional discourse in a society whose language and culture do not support such emotional manifestations. Inadvertently, they helped propel artistic disciplines into the educational system, which have been scarce and poor quality thus far. Students react with evident yearning and delight. The particularity and advantage of arts therapy within a collectivistic society have become clearer as an indirect and metaphorical method of treatment, which has proven to be especially appropriate culturally, for clients and families in a traditional society.

Dwairy (2015) defined a form of therapy that could replace psychoanalysis, which he terms *culture analysis*: "An analysis within the self-representations of the culture. It is aimed at helping the client revise his or her belief system and manage it differently in order to cope better with various life situations" (p. 49). Dwairy describes how the exploration of intrapsychic conflict in therapy can be replaced by an intra-cultural exploration of the client's own culture. He recommends that therapists apply aspects of the client's culture in a way that challenges the client's unilateral understanding of his/her hardships. Only then can therapist and client progress beyond the client's defensiveness and support a better adaptation to the community. This treatment is based on metaphors arising from the client's verbal statements, associated phrases, culture-based idioms and similes. As such, it is particularly suitable for arts-based therapeutic interventions.

Much can be learned by inquiring into the evolution of arts therapy in Arab public education in Israel. In the beginning there was extensive efforts at public *relations*. Arts therapists presented both the nature of the new profession and its benefits for students, families and school staff. New languages had to be encountered: the language of Western art, the language of Western psychology and undeniably also the therapeutic language which is very different from the educational language familiar to school staff.

Whereas in the first ten years after introducing arts therapy into the educational system, most therapists working in Arab society were Jewish; nowadays the vast majority come from Arab society itself. This profound change came about through *top-down* pressure from faculty members in training programs and field supervisors who sought to train the ever-growing numbers of IPA arts therapists. This was complemented by a *bottom-up* process where school staff and families of clients realized the potential of the new discipline and engaged in it alongside their Jewish counterparts, thus taking growing responsibility over less advantaged members of the IPA society.

Initially, as students or in practicum, each therapist inadvertently became a *representative* of Israeli Arab society to her peers-in-training. In recent years, the number of students in arts therapy programs hailing from Arab society has grown, and they now serve as a support group for one another. Each and every therapist has to make a profound and personal journey into the domains of Western art and therapy. This entails facing numerous feminist issues that challenge cultural perceptions of her role and destiny as a woman. When working in their communities, they serve as emissaries of perspectives that value both individual needs and the familial and communal context. They serve as role models for their clients, their families and their co-workers at school by embodying the potential for change through the therapeutic process. Although mothers first approached therapy as a means of securing treatment for their children, they soon began seeking treatment for themselves as well. Fathers are also much more involved in their child's therapy, and are inclined to take an equal part in parental guidance when called upon to make necessary changes at home. Thus, therapists have become agents of change, encouraging gradual changes in the way women and children are perceived in a closed and traditional society.

This particular example of gradual infiltration of arts therapy into Israeli Arab society demonstrates the feasibility of integrating therapy in other countries struggling with a complex social fabric, whether stemming from an active conflict between ethnic, cultural and/or religious groups, or from a historic conflict such as in the cases of a colonial regime, slavery or settlers who have driven off an indigenous people. The authors suggest that culturally sensitive arts therapy, particularly when applied within a public and inclusive educational system, can affect both students and their families in an optimal way. It is our belief that Jewish and Arab therapists working in Arab society can aspire towards *cultural proficiency*, setting aside biases discrimination and a sense of superiority:

> Knowledge about the Other is truly an impossibility on two counts. Ontologically, otherness is precisely that which defies our own sameness and exists in a relation of exteriority to the self...when I think I know, when I think I understand the Other, I am exercising my knowledge over the Other, shrouding the Other in my own totality. The

> Other becomes an object of my comprehension, my world, my narrative, reducing the Other to me... Insofar as I can be receptive and susceptible, I can learn from the Other as one who is absolutely different from myself.
>
> (Todd, 2003, p. 15)

And Finally, a Personal Note on the Shared Process of Writing This Chapter

From the very beginning, it has been clear this chapter should be written as a team process between an Arab and a Jew. Our interaction created a total that is greater than its parts. Each had a chance to learn attentively and impartially how best to observe the culture and perceptions of her own culture through the eyes of her colleague, and vice versa. It is our belief that the transitional language of arts therapy encouraged our efforts. As such, it may become the chosen path to helping children and adults from Arab and Jewish societies to have a growth-promoting, compassionate and secure engagement.

Acknowledgments

We would like to thank our dear families: Zakiah's parents Khalil and Aida, who supported her unusual choice of vocation and believe in her professional development, as well as her spouse Bassem and her children Youssef, Ahmad and Samara. We are grateful to Yael's parents Michael and Ofra, who paved the way to art therapy in Israel, as well as her spouse Eran and son Yotam, who advised and helped with the translation and proofreading of this chapter.

References

Abu Baker, K. (2008). Welfare, modernism and tradition: How Palestinian women in Israel cope with changes in their life framework. In R. Gharra & A. Manna (Eds.), *Arab society 2: Population, society, economy* (pp. 359–384). Jerusalem: Van Leer Institute and Hakibbutz Hameuchad Publishing House. [Hebrew].

Abu Baker, K., & Dwairy, M. (2003). Cultural norms versus state law in treating incest: A suggested model for Arab families. *Child Abuse & Neglect*, *27*, 109–123.

Abu-Saad, I. (2004). Separate and unequal: The role of the state educational system in maintaining the subordination of Israel's Palestinian Arab citizens. *Social Identities*, *10*, 101–127. https://doi.org/10.1080/1350463042000191010

Ahmed, S.H., & Siddiqi, M.N. (2006). Healing through art therapy in disaster settings. *Lancet*, *368*, S28–S29.

Al-Haj, M. (1989). Social research on family lifestyles among Arabs in Israel. *Journal of Comparative Family Studies*, *20*(2), 175–195.

Al-Haj, M. (1995). *Education, empowerment and control: The case of the Arabs in Israel*. New York: State University of New York Press.

Al-Krenawi, A., & Graham, J.R. (2011). Mental health help-seeking among Arab university students in Israel, differentiated by religion. *Mental Health, Religion & Culture 14*(2), 157–167.

American Art Therapy Association. (2013). *Ethical principles for art therapists*. Retrieved from: https://arttherapy.org/wp-content/uploads/2017/06/Ethical-Principles-for-Art-Therapists.pdf

Angel, T. (2014). *"How Much Can a Bridge Carry?" An analysis of the life stories of the Arab Israeli citizen bibliotherapists in Israel*. Dissertation for the degree of Doctor of Philosophy, University of Sussex, UK.

Arar, K.H., & Abu-Rabia-Queder, S. (2011). Turning points in the lives of two pioneer Arab women principals in Israel. *Gender and Education*, *23*(4), 415–429.

Awais, Y.J., & Yali, A.M. (2013). A call for diversity: The need to recruit and retain ethnic minority students in art therapy. *Art Therapy: Journal of the American Art Therapy Association*, *30*(3), 130–134.

Behrens, G.A. (2019). *Use of traditional and nontraditional instruments with traumatized children in Bethlehem, West Bank*. Retrieved from: https://academic.oup.com/mtp/article-abstract/30/2/196/1138838

Central Bureau of Statistics (2018). *Israel in figures*. Retrieved from: https://www.cbs.gov.il/he/publications/doclib/2018/shnatonnew

Chilcote, R.T. (2007). Art therapy with child tsunami survivors in Sri Lanka. *Art Therapy*, *24*(4), 156–162.

Daoud, N., Sergienko, R., O'Campo, P., & Shoham-Vardi, I. (2017). Disorganization theory neighborhood social capital, and ethnic inequalities in intimate partner violence between Arab and Jewish women citizens of Israel. *Journal of Urban Health*, *94*, 648–665. https://doi.org/10.1007/s11524-017-0196-4

Dror Hadar, D. (2015). *"Autobiography": An educational program for the promotion of Arab women students' self-efficacy and self-expression*. Doctorate thesis for the University of Faculty of Babes – Bolyai: Psychology and Educational Sciences, Cluj-Napoca, Rumania.

Dwairy, A.M. (1998). *Cross-cultural counseling: The Arab-palestinian case*. New York: The Haworth Press.

Dwairy, M. (2002). Foundations of psychosocial dynamic personality theory of collective people. *Clinical Psychology Review*, *22*, 343–360.

Dwairy, M. (2015). *From psycho-analysis to culture-analysis: A within-culture psychotherapy*. Hampshire: Palgrave Macmillan.

Dwairy, M., & Van Sickle, D.T. (1996). Western psychotherapy in traditional Arabic societies. *Clinical Psychology Review*, *16*(3), 231–249.

Haen, C. (2007). "Make me wanna holler": Dramatic encounters with boys from the inner city. In V.A. Camilleri (Ed.), *Healing the Inner City child: Creative arts therapies with at-risk youth* (pp. 212–228). Philadelphia, PA: Jessica Kingsley.

Institution for Social Security (2015). *Poverty indicators and social inequalities: Annual report for 2014*. Jerusalem: Institution for Social Security.

Kristeva J. (1991). *Strangers to ourselves*. New York: Columbia University Press.

Landy, R.J. (2008). *The couch and the stage: Integrating words and action in psychotherapy*. Plymouth: Jason Aronson.

Massarwa, Z. (2016). *The experience of art therapists from the Arab society when facing mandatory reporting on child abuse*. MA thesis. University of Haifa, Faculty of Social Welfare and Health sciences, School of Creative Arts Therapies.

McNiff, S., & Barlow, G.C. (2009). Cross-cultural psychotherapy and art. *Art Therapy*, *26*(3), 100–106.

Moodley, R., & Walcott R. (Eds.). (2010). *Counseling across and beyond cultures: Exploring the works of Clemont E. Vontress in clinical practice*. Toronto: University of Toronto Press.

Potash, J.S., Doby-Copeland, C., Stepney, S.A., Washington, B.N., Vance, L.D., Short, G.M., … Ballbé ter Maat, M. (2015). Advancing multicultural and diversity competence in art therapy: American Art Therapy Association Multicultural Committee 1990–2015. *Art Therapy*, *32*(3), 146–150.

Quinlan, R., Schweitzer, R.D., Khawaja, N., & Griffin, J. (2015). Psychotherapy evaluation of a school-based creative arts therapy programme for adolescents from refugee backgrounds. *The Arts in Psychotherapy*, *47*, 72–78.

Qur'an 49:13 (2013). translated by Abdullah Yusuf Ali. Ware, Hertfordshire: Wordsworth Editions Limited.

Robb, M. (2002). Beyond the orphanages: Art therapy with Russian children. *Art Therapy*, *19*(4), 146–150.

Roth-Yaniv, S., Mayan, Y., & Hazut, T. (1999). Preliminary aspects of a triangular encounter: Art, culture and therapy through the arts in the Druze sector in Israel. *Issues in Special Education & Inclusion*, *14*(1), 105–114. [Hebrew].

Sideris, J. (2017). From you and me to us and we. *Children Australia*, *42*(2), 79–86.

Smooha, S. (2018). How do western democracies cope with the challenge of societal diversity? *Nations and Nationalism*, *24*(2), 215–236.

Snir, S., Regev, D., Keinan, V., Abd El Kader-Shahada, H., Salamey, A., Mekel, D., … Alkara, M. (2018). Art therapy in the Israeli education system–a qualitative meta-analysis. *International Journal of Art Therapy*, *23*(4), 169–179.

Srour, R. (2015). Transference and countertransference issues during times of violent political conflict: The Arab therapist–Jewish patient dyad. *Clinical Social Work Journal*, *43*, 407–418.

Sue, D.W., & Sue, D. (1999). *Counseling the culturally different: Theory and practice*. New York: John Wiley.

Talwar, S. (2015). Culture, diversity, and identity: From margins to center. *Art Therapy*, *32*(3), 100–103.

Talwar, S., Iyer, J., & Doby-Copeland, C. (2004). The invisible veil: Changing paradigms in the art therapy profession. *Art therapy*, *21*(1), 44–48.

Todd, S. (2003). *Learning from the other: Levinas, psychoanalysis and ethical possibilities in education*. New York: State University of New York Press.

U.S. Commission on Civil Rights Briefing Report (2010). *The educational effectiveness of historically black colleges and universities*. Washington, DC. https://files.eric.ed.gov/fulltext/ED513988.pdf

Vardimon, S. (2011). *Touch the elephant: On a seminar on the subject of the Jewish-Arab meeting in the treatment room* (Hebrew). Retrieved August 30, 2020 from: http://www.hebpsy.net/articles.asp?id=2678

Zoabi, K., & Savaya, R. (2015). Cultural identity and intervention strategies of Arab social workers in Israel. *Journal of Society and Welfare*, *35*, 397–421. (Hebrew).

Part II

Specific Working Models in the Education System

6 Parent-child Art Psychotherapy in the Education System

Dafna Regev and Rona Tamir

Introduction

Over the past few years, the literature in the field of parent-child art psychotherapy has grown considerably. This field is particularly suitable for working with young children as it extends the influence of therapy by working closely with parents. Creative expression in art therapy enables both the child and the parent to produce spontaneous artwork channeling emotions, unconscious fears, wishes, fantasies and memories which can be harnessed to strengthen the parent-child relationship.

Parent-child art psychotherapy in the Israeli educational system has developed on two concurrent axes. On the one hand, over the years, more arts therapists have been integrated into the education system and have started working with children as young as kindergarten. On the other, advances in the field of parent-child art psychotherapy have prompted growing numbers of arts therapists who recognize the value and effectiveness of this model to train as parent-child therapists. The next step was to make parent-child art psychotherapy available in the education system for clients whose parents are willing to come to kindergarten or school on a regular basis to participate in their child's therapeutic hour. This chapter discusses the impact of parent-child art psychotherapy and describes the ways it is applied in the Israeli education system.

Theoretical Background

Parent-child Psychotherapy

In parent-child psychotherapy, the parent and child work together in the therapy room, and the focus of therapy is the parent-child relationship. This model is based on theories positing that a good parent-child relationship promotes optimal child development (Winnicott, 1971) such as attachment theory (Bowlby, 1979), object relations theory (Mahler, Pine, & Bergman, 1975) and family therapy theories (Minuchin, 2007). There are many parent-child psychotherapy models, each of which ascribes a slightly different role to the psychotherapist. However, in all models, the goal of therapy is to improve the interactions and the relationship between parent and child, and all require the presence of one parent, and occasionally both parents, in the therapy room.

In this chapter we focus on the model developed by the late Miriam Ben-Aaron and her colleagues (Ben-Aaron et al., 2001; Harel et al., 2006; Kaplan et al., 2010). The model is mentalization-based (Fonagy, Gergely, & Target, 2007) within a relational psychoanalytic orientation and is designed to treat relationship disorders during childhood. It is based on the acknowledgment of the complexity of parenthood and the processes of change that occur in parents. It aims to provide a deeper understanding of the dynamics of intergenerational transferences of psychopathological representations and their prevention. It starts from the premise that children develop unique relationships with each parent and that children need the active involvement of both parents in their lives. It also attributes crucial importance to the developmental contexts in which the child is raised and is sensitive to the difficulties that can arise in child development as a result of the nature of the relationship. Therapy consists of a mother-child, father-child meeting every alternating week with the same psychotherapist. Every two or three weeks, the psychotherapist also meets with the parents for parental guidance without the presence of the child. The presence of the child with his/her parents in therapy may initiate tensions and conflicts from the very beginning of the therapeutic process, which can catalyze changes in their relationship. The psychotherapist helps to elicit issues that are both implicit and explicit. The psychotherapist supports the reflective function of the members of the dyad, where the new experiences and behaviors create new representations of the relationship. The development of parents' reflective thinking during parental guidance develops their ability to mentalize and creates a safe space that contributes to the success of therapy.

Parent-child Art Psychotherapy in the Education System

The parent-child art psychotherapy model combines parent-child psychotherapy with art therapy. In this model, both the work process and the art product are considered to encourage meaningful mental processes (Gavron, 2013). The model invites the parent and child to participate in a visual and creative experience that uses the imagination and enables non-verbal, symbolic expression while engaging in an artistic activity that adults and children do together (Proulx, 2003). It also fosters the development of mutual recognition between parents and their children which is facilitated through the artwork and its specific support processes (Gavron, 2013). One of the distinctive features of parent-child art psychotherapy is the art therapist's provision of a rich variety of different artistic materials and techniques to the dyad according to the developmental stage of the child, while at the same time allowing the parent to experience the artwork in a way that is symbolically and mentally appropriate for him/her. Occasionally the parents' tangible encounters with their artwork allow them to translate and interpret conscious and unconscious meaningful content into words. The inclusion of artistic creation as part of the therapeutic process provides a specific response to the two goals of parent-child psychotherapy: the fostering of an interpersonal interaction as a space for change and the invitation to the dyad to observe and examine internal representations.

Over the last two decades, clinical work in parent-child art psychotherapy has evolved, and gradually, research and literature in the field has emerged in several countries including Israel. In Canada, two books on parent-child art psychotherapy have been published (Prooulx, 2003, 2017) and a dissertation on this subject has also been written (Dancette-De Bresson, 2016). In England, researchers Taylor, Beck and colleagues (2013) reviewed the changes in the field of art therapy and found that 50%–70% of all art therapists working with children and adolescents involve parents or other significant figures in the child's life in this therapy. In addition, a large section of a book on art therapy with young children in England was devoted entirely to parent-child art psychotherapy (Meyerowitz-Katz & Reddick, 2017). In North Korea, several articles have been published on parent-child art psychotherapy and parental guidance (Kynng, Doctrol, Choi, & Park, 2016). In Israel, a number of researchers have published theoretical and empirical work (Gavron, 2013, 2017; Markman Zinemanas, 1994; Regev & Snir, 2014, 2015, 2017).

In the last decade, parent-child art psychotherapy has begun to be integrated into kindergartens and school settings. Parents are integrated into the therapeutic process to facilitate the promotion of emotional, social and educational goals in the child's educational setting as part of a holistic approach that combines therapy with education (Shapira, 2018). In a recent study (Tamir & Regev, 2020), we examined the therapeutic encounter between client and parents by reviewing 136 therapy follow-up diary entries (including diary entries that were written following parental guidance sessions) that were filled out by four art therapists working in public primary and special education schools. These therapists were involved in five different parent-child art psychotherapies for an entire academic year and documented the processes in their semi-structured diary entries every week at the end of the therapy session. The following section outlines the content that emerged from these diary entries and illustrates the ways in which these art therapists implemented the parent-child art psychotherapy model. We present examples reflective of many different clients treated over the years which thus do not represent one specific client.

Description of the Working Model and Clinical Examples

Goals

Art therapists who work according to the parent-child art psychotherapy model in the educational system set several goals for these treatments. The first is to acquire a better understanding of the client's family environment.

This involves understanding the family dynamics and its impact on the student. By contrast to the limited acquaintance with students' families in general in the education system, the parent-child art psychotherapy model and the frequent meetings with parents provide the student and his/her family with more extensive care, including parental guidance. The second goal is to improve the relationship between the parent and the child, based on the assumption that enhancing the relationship will contribute to the child's functioning and behavior in other relationships, including with peers and the educational staff. The third goal is to improve the client's functioning. This involves developing the student's level of independence, boosting self-image, improving communication, dealing with anxiety and improving management of life transitions. The fourth goal relates to improving the parents' functioning and their ability to support their son or daughter on his/her own path. This involves developing the parents' mentalization and listening skills, empowering them and enabling their understanding of what their child is feeling. These goals can only be achieved within an optimal and contained relationship with the art therapist.

The following example demonstrates how the therapeutic goals can change during the therapeutic process. These goals relate to the therapeutic relationship between the student, the parents and the art therapist, and to the broader relationship with the educational system. Seven-year-old Yoav experienced a great deal of turmoil after starting kindergarten and his problems worsened in first grade. Yoav spoke very little, expressed a lack of interest in general and in school, and often had an angry expression and tended to gaze downward. It was clear that he was experiencing stress about everything that was going on around him and physically responded to authority figures who approached him. Most of his time was spent outside the classroom in the field or yard. During a conversation with Yoav's parents, a different picture emerged. They described their family of five children. Yoav was the youngest, and they portrayed him as a curious and sweet boy who was sociable and communicative with his siblings and extended family. According to them, he was a loving and embracing child, a "prince" whose parents helped him whenever he found things difficult to do (from showering, dressing and serving him food in front of the television). His parents found it hard to believe that their child was aggressive and uncooperative at school. Consequently, it was decided to refer the family to parent-child art psychotherapy at school. The process consisted of three main stages. The goal of the first stage was to build trust and create a therapeutic relationship between Yoav, his parents and the art therapist in the therapy room as well as to strengthen the parents' relationship with the educational staff, with the art therapist acting as an intermediary.

During this stage, there was a dramatic improvement in Yoav's behavior in the school setting, as well as in his level of openness to learning and his relationships with the educational staff. There was also a significant improvement in his parents' relationship with the educational and therapeutic staff. Trust was established and a program was defined that included changes in the parents' behavior during their interactions with Yoav at home.

The second stage involved the therapeutic goal of monitoring the situation at home. It became clear that Yoav's behavior was undergoing a change. He became cheeky, started fighting with his siblings, broke things, went wild and often expressed frustration and anger towards his parents. His parents were surprised and struggled to cope with the change in his behavior and adhere to the parental guidance program. At the same time, the chaos at home also manifested in the art therapy room during the parent-child art psychotherapy sessions with each of Yoav's parents. During the session with his mother, Yoav drew a picture of a blockaded sealed-off house. When asked about his artwork, he became withdrawn. However, in the session with his father, Yoav talked about his mother's verbal aggressions. Yoav's sharing of this information during the session in the presence of his father facilitated change and a more authentic and direct commitment on behalf of his parents during parental guidance sessions. Listening to the parents describe their distress, as well as empowering them, helped the parents understand what Yoav was going through and his mother's aggression stopped.

In the third stage of therapy, the goal was to improve the parent-child relationship to foster Yoav's functioning and behavior within other relationships, including with his peers and the educational staff. In terms of the educational setting, there was a deterioration in his behavior in the classroom, but even though Yoav was agitated, he was not aggressive. He would leave the classroom but soon returned. Yoav was able to identify and express his feelings, felt less intimidated and gradually became more open to his schoolwork and to socializing with his peers. In addition, he became more independent and less reliant on his parents. The parental guidance sessions were expanded to help his parents strengthen and maintain the changes. This example suggests that in the education system, changing therapeutic goals often addresses both the therapeutic relationship and improvement in the student's functioning in the system.

The Therapeutic Setting

The therapeutic setting in parent-child art psychotherapy involves the continuous participation of parents in the therapy sessions with their children. When this occurs within the education system, the parents need to come to school during their working hours, which may be impossible for some families. Thus, this model is not suitable for all families but only for those who can commit to attending regular sessions at school. There are situations where, due to the therapeutic work within the educational system, it is necessary to create a specific setting for each family. The following example illustrates such a case and highlights issues relating to each client's ability to deal with the challenges of the therapeutic setting.

Jasmine, a seven-year-old student, looked like a fairy. She wandered around the corridors and school yard, walked around during lessons and spun her own dreams and stories. From time to time, she would sit down in different places to play with dolls which she brought from home. She seemed only partially aware of the need to enter the classroom. After a very turbulent year in first grade, the staff recommended she be given parent-child art psychotherapy at school. Because of the high demands of the parents' workplaces and their roles as senior managers, and after many mutual discussions, a fixed setting was arranged. The mother attended the session once every two weeks during the first school period and then went to her work and the father attended once every three weeks during his lunch break. The parental guidance sessions were also scheduled at special times to suit both parents. The question arose as to whether Jasmine could deal with this complex setting and still experience the sense of continuity and consistency she needed in the therapeutic process given her lack of awareness of time or continuity. Surprisingly, Jasmine remembered and even reminded her parents and the art therapist who was supposed to attend the session each week. This example demonstrates the complexity of adapting the therapy setting to the parents' availability and the student's ability to tolerate changes to the setting.

The diary study suggested that despite the parents' goodwill, there were instances in which they failed to attend sessions or had no other choice but to bring another child with them to the sessions (for example, in the case of a sibling's illness), which made them less than fully available for the parent-child art psychotherapy session. This situation often led to a lack of clarity about therapy and constituted a challenge in terms of not knowing who would be attending the session with the student. As a result, there were sessions when the student attended therapy without his/her parents. These specific sessions were problematic for the art therapists since they had prepared for parent-child art psychotherapy and suddenly found themselves obligated to treat the student alone. In a private clinic, these types of session would possibly have been canceled, but in the public sector the therapeutic work continues under existing conditions. Importantly, when children in parent-child art psychotherapy learn that their parents cannot attend a session, they may develop a feeling of immense disappointment since they look forward to the parents' attendance and want to spend time with them.

The following example illustrates the challenges involved when one parent cannot attend a session at school. Ten-year-old Shachar was receiving parent-child art psychotherapy with his parents at school. The sessions were structured to accommodate the parents' schedule: his mother was present three sessions in a row and his father came to a regular session once a month, followed by a parental guidance session. The art therapy focused on the issue of separation in the symbiotic relationship that Shachar had formed with his mother. As therapy progressed, there appeared to be an improvement in separation, but at the same time, the mother began to exhibit various signs of strain, fatigue, shortness of breath, and she complained about the smell of the art materials and had a hard time being in the art therapy room. One morning, the mother sent an SMS to the art therapist that she would not be coming to the session and informed Shachar at home. Shachar came to the art therapy session alone, but throughout the session he seemed embarrassed, shifted uncomfortably in his chair, appeared more withdrawn, bit his nails and barely spoke or looked up. Shachar drew a picture of an egg starting to hatch and repeatedly inquired when the session would be over. His difficulty dealing with intimacy and the current situation was tangible, but through the creative work, the art therapist observed gradual signs of change and separation that emerged in connection with his mother. During a session a week later, Shachar expressed his anger at his mother's decision not to come to the art therapy session and he asked his parents to attend them regularly. This case study demonstrates the complexity of individual therapy sessions that occur when parents do not attend. However, since the overall goal is to promote the student's functioning, many art therapists often find other ways to further promote students during these sessions.

Art therapists applying the parent-child art psychotherapy model in the education system often work in rooms that have been re-arranged and adapted for therapy. Sometimes they create specific spaces in the room that enable the parent and child to work together. The setting of the art therapy room can be tailored specifically to the parent-child sessions, unlike the school setting, with its educational activities, school trips, ceremonies and events that interfere every so often with the preferred therapy sequence and structure. The findings here suggested that the art therapists made significant attempts to maintain the continuity of therapy, especially in parent-child art psychotherapy sessions involving the presence of parents. Perhaps they felt that the parents' efforts to attend these sessions should be matched by efforts on the part of the system providing the service, as well as their own efforts to hold the weekly sessions. To do so, the art therapists sometimes changed their work schedules or changed the length of a session to accommodate parent-child art psychotherapy sessions as continuously as possible.

The following example illustrates how school activities are integrated into the therapeutic work and occasionally influence the course of therapy. Gilad, an 11-year-old, experienced a deterioration in his emotional state following his parents' separation and his father's departure from their home. In the first phase, his father continued to attend the sessions, but approximately a month later he asked to stop. The changes in the setting were difficult for Gilad. His father's decision to stop attending the parent-child art psychotherapy sessions coincided with the period of annual ceremonies at school (several national memorial days), all of which occurred on the day of his scheduled therapy and specifically during his therapy hour. Although the art therapist changed the treatment schedule to accommodate Gilad and his mother, the change in the setting intensified Gilad's feelings of distress and he found it difficult to persist and attend art therapy. On one occasion, his mother got to school during a ceremony and waited for Gilad, but he refused to go into the art therapy room. The therapy sessions resumed normally one month later, Gilad returned to art therapy and gradually worked through his distress over the family crisis and the changes in his life. This example details the complexity of finding the appropriate time and place for art therapy when dealing with both the system and family constraints. This complex situation demands flexibility on the part of the art therapist.

In the parent-child art psychotherapy model and its variants, there are usually clear standards as to the specific number of parent-child sessions and parental guidance sessions. Within the education system, adjustments need to be made to adapt to the needs of each family and respective clients. For example, for approximately half of the parental guidance sessions that were evaluated in this study, the parents were able to come together as a couple, but in the second half of the year, due to difficulties in the spousal relationship, the parental guidance sessions were held separately for each parent. Towards the end of the academic year, there is occasionally an increase in the parents' need for parental guidance, which may lead to an increase in their frequency. The following example illustrates a case in which the mother attended the parental guidance sessions alone. In Gilad's case (mentioned above), his refusal to attend the therapy sessions led to a period of approximately a month during which the mother attended parental guidance sessions instead of the parent-child art psychotherapy sessions. Initially, since the mother felt she was being criticized by her family and children for her role in her husband's departure from the home, she focused on basic survival issues and needs and found it difficult to allocate her reserves and extra energy to observe her relationship with Gilad. During the parental guidance process, a mental space was slowly created that allowed her to expand her reflective thinking ability about the parent-child art psychotherapy process with Gilad. She realized that during these encounters in the months since the family crisis occurred, her attentiveness to Gilad's needs had been mainly focused on his basic physiological needs (such as food and sleep). This realization within the parental guidance setting, along with the intervention of the art therapist, enabled her to set new goals that included improving her interactions with Gilad, as well as thinking about other ways she could support him. This case highlights the need for flexibility and adaptation for each family situation.

Characteristics of the Parent-Child Interaction

Art therapists working according to the parent-child art psychotherapy model in the educational system encourage the parent and child to connect and communicate with one another. The diary entries clearly indicated that in each session there was an eagerness to work on the relationship which was expressed in their behavior, such as sitting in close proximity to one another or having physical contact during the session, creating a joint drawing, and playing and speaking about things together. In most of the sessions that were documented in the diary entries, parents related to their children with considerable patience, attentiveness, motivation, openness and a willingness to establish their relationship. In the art therapy room, the children expressed their desire for playfulness, liveliness, initiative and creativity that led to connections with their parents. At the same time, the entries showed that in many sessions there were difficulties during their interactions that included resistance, rejection, communication difficulties, criticism and differences between what each participant wanted from the session. These difficulties also surfaced in the parental guidance sessions between the parents and the art therapists.

During these sessions, the entries often indicated that there was a need for one of the members of the dyad (most often the child) to achieve separation, which was expressed in various ways such as physical distance, disregard for the other member, the desire to work alone, lack of participation in shared conversations and others. At its core, the individual's natural need for separation does not necessarily represent a difficulty in a relationship but can be viewed as a developmental stage in which the child expands his/her level of independence and separation from the parent. The participants' interpretation or management of the need for separation could lead to situations in which it was possible to continue the interaction compared to situations in which this need led to difficulties in the relationship. The following example shows how a daughter's need for separation from her father was reconciled in the presence of the art therapist. Zohar was six years old when she was referred to parent-child art psychotherapy at school. She behaved childishly, was often angry, offended and then would become withdrawn during difficult times. Her parents were at odds with each other, so the therapy sessions were held alternatively with each of them, and the parental guidance sessions were scheduled immediately after the art therapy session for each of them individually. In a session with Zohar and her father, they created a drawing of space using gouache paints. This subject was dear to them both, as Zohar's father had chosen her name (which signifies brightness and radiance) because of his love for the heavens and the stars. By engaging in a subject that connected the father and daughter, the artwork created a great deal of intimacy between them. At one point when they were drawing the stars, the father started correcting and criticizing Zohar's work. She got terribly angry, refused to continue, moved away from her father and became withdrawn and refused to respond, answer or create anything for a few minutes. Her extreme reaction to the insult was much like her usual behavior with her father, but this time, with the help of the art therapist, her father managed to connect with her and return to the joint drawing together.

In general, and specifically in the educational framework, short-term processes of change and development within the parent-child relationships can be observed during parent-child art psychotherapy. These changes are facilitated by systemic work while the parents are present in therapy and within the framework of therapy in the educational system. The changes in the parent-child relationship can be manifested in several ways. The first is in the way the parent and child are seated, their physical contact and proximity. It can be seen in the way they express themselves, their shared humor which sometimes develops during the sessions and conversations that become more meaningful as the members of the dyad persevere in therapy. It can also be observed in the creative processes where they start to use similar art materials, choose images after a process of collective thinking and oftentimes work together on a shared format. As therapy lasts for approximately half the academic year, the reflective ability that both the parent and gradually the student develop become more apparent.

The following example illustrates how sessions that commenced with many interaction challenges evolved during the therapeutic process and were characterized at a later stage by improved openness in the relationship. Ten-year-old Nadav was referred to parent-child art psychotherapy at school on the basis of reports from the staff about his emotional distress, crying, loneliness and inability to engage in schoolwork and social interactions. During the intake session which took place in the presence of both parents, it emerged that the parents were involved in a serious relationship crisis. In the first few sessions, it was evident that Nadav desperately wanted and needed a relationship with his father, but the father rejected him both verbally and behaviorally and humiliated him over his disabilities. Consequently, a parental guidance session was scheduled for the father alone. The art therapist shared her experience with the father, expressing empathy about the difficulty of raising a child with learning disabilities, but at the same time she refused to collaborate with the father's approach towards his son. The conversation brought up many "ghosts" (Fraiberg, Adelson, & Shapiro, 1975) from the father's difficult and estranged childhood. The father grew up as a single son of Holocaust survivor parents who separated in a complicated divorce. Nadav's father, who lived with his mother, experienced his own father's humiliation and anger towards him and severed ties with him. The father's realization that he was recreating this in his behavior towards his son allowed the father to recognize his physical difficulties in embracing his son and even looking at him in a positive light. That same year, Nadav's father learned to express his affection towards his son more spontaneously and was even impressed by his thriving creative abilities. This case exemplifies how observing the relationship with parents during the parent-child art psychotherapy process enabled a significant change in the relationship and subsequently in the student's functioning at school.

The Art Therapist's Position in Parent-Child Art Psychotherapy

The art therapist provides the container and facilitates the relationship between parent and child. Typically, the students in art therapy form a relationship very quickly with the art therapist, which includes pursuing physical proximity, eye contact, requests for technical assistance, verbal sharing and sharing in the artwork or in play. In addition, the art therapist's relationship with the parents develops during their collaborative work. The diary entries mentioned how parents learned to ask for the therapist's support and thoughts on issues that concerned them, and sought advice on their parenting styles and how to conduct themselves in situations where they felt unsure about how to interact with their children. In this study, the relationship with the art therapist was only described as ambivalent in a few cases and the members of the dyad seemed to experience both a desire for and difficulties with the relationship in the same session. The following example shows how rapidly the transference relationship between the client's mother and the art therapist was created. Ten-year-old Yoav and his mother arrived late for their joint parent-child art psychotherapy session. Instead of apologizing, the mother asked the art therapist: "Where do you buy your clothes?" The art therapist hesitated and was surprised by the direct question and tried to understand its intent. The mother told the art therapist that she reminded her of her mother. She mentioned that because of her mother's disability, she would often buy clothes for her and this why she inquired about the art therapist's attire. The connection between the art therapist and the grandmother, the mother's mother, was linked to the representation of the "good grandmother" (an idea proposed by Daniel Stern, 1995, 1998) which was experienced by the members of the dyad in therapy and recurred later in the process.

A variety of interventions have been developed to better enable the art therapist to support parent and child. These intervention techniques are described below.

Interventions that structure the setting. These interventions help the art therapist structure the complex therapeutic setting that involves students' parents in the educational system. Occasionally, these include interventions that are intended to deal with issues such as who will attend and when the sessions will be held. They include interventions that guide members of the dyad to engage in certain activities in the art therapy room, such as art making. The hustle and bustle of the school setting means that a variety of outside stimuli can be heard in the art therapy room. Art therapists are often concerned about what constitutes the "right" amount of "outside" input should be allowed to affect the events in the art therapy room and when or why it is appropriate to allow outsiders into the therapy room that violate the boundaries of the "setting" (such as when students invite their home room teachers to view their artworks). The following example shows how the entry or exit of the parents and child from the school art therapy room can often result in encounters with other students or staff members, which sometimes influence the therapeutic process. As mentioned above, Gilad had been dealing with his father's absence from home. One morning on his way to art therapy with his mother, the music teacher met them in the corridor and told Gilad's mother about an issue that came up in her last lesson with him. Gilad was quiet during their encounter, but in the therapy room he exploded and expressed great emotional intensity. The feeling was that the encounter and conversation outside the art therapy room triggered Gilad to collectively perceive the music teacher (who complained about him), his mother (whom he accused of causing his father to leave) and the art therapist as a female coalition he needed to combat. In subsequent sessions, his drawings dealt with battlegrounds and fortified trenches where soldiers were fighting. This case illustrates the complex challenge of separating the therapy setting from the outside world in the education setting and specifically when parents are involved in the process.

Interventions and exercises in art and play. In most parent-child art psychotherapy sessions, art therapists offer and assist the parent and child to actively participate in creative work or play. Depending on the goal of the session, the art therapist presents appropriate creative materials, suggests or models collaborative or individual creative work techniques and at times serves as an auxiliary ego for clients. During the parents' guidance sessions, the art therapist also occasionally introduces creative processes. This can involve observing joint artworks from the parent-child sessions or starting a new artwork. At times this can be a joint drawing by both parents which can help them observe their relationship with their child. The following example shows how the shared creative space of the parent and child helped foster the student's emotional expression and processing of experiences. Seven-year-old Matan and his mother drew an aquarium during a parent-child art psychotherapy session at school (inspired by Lucille Proulx's technique, 2003). By drawing many air bubbles, Matan managed to articulate his sense of choking that he experiences when his parents quarrel at home.

Interventions that broaden emotional understanding. Art therapists often use reflection of the emotional state of the members of the dyad to expand their vocabulary and their understanding of their feelings and that of their partner during a session. In the parental guidance sessions, the art therapists reflect and interpret the parents' feelings through text and creativity to help them connect their childhood experiences with their emotions that emerge and influence their relationships with their child. Now and again, the use of questions can help to broaden the observations, emotional understanding and connections between content that surfaces during parent-child art psychotherapy sessions and events from client's real world. The following example shows how parental guidance can help broaden the parents' perceptions of their emotional states and relationships with their children. Five-year-old Yaron attended parent-child art psychotherapy sessions in a kindergarten setting following a domestic accident in which he fell off a couch and had a concussion. His parents were relatively older immigrants who often came to the therapy sessions in the morning after their night shifts working in a factory and usually arrived tired, passive and downhearted. During their parental guidance sessions, the parents described their feeling of guilt, concern and fear about what happened to Yaron, as well as their fear that he could be injured again because of his tendency to run wild at home combined with their exhaustion in bringing up Yaron and his younger brother. The art therapist chose to use the parental guidance sessions to inquire about the mother's nickname for Yaron, and she learned that it was her father's name, Yaron's grandfather. He had committed suicide when Yaron's mother was Yaron's age. The mother's ability to reveal her early childhood pain helped both her and Yaron's father to understand the source of panic they experienced when Yaron was injured and the need to define a behavioral framework in the home that was appropriate for their children's developmental stages and need for movement and play. The parents' process in these sessions helped them to understand their parenthood more extensively. Often the use of art-based interventions in parental guidance can also help.

Parent-child relationship interventions. This intervention is designed to help the members of the dyad improve their relationship. It can include attempts to help a parent praise his/her child and contain the content and emotions that this evokes. It also includes reflection and verbal interpretation by the art therapist about events that have occurred in the therapy room and occasionally behavioral intervention techniques to help members of the dyad connect with each other. The following example illustrates how the art therapist enabled a parent to help his child. Gili, a nine year old, came to a session with his father and created a hospital using clay, stating that sick people had been hospitalized and his father was the doctor. The father, who was not a doctor at all, was surprised and found it difficult to create anything and sat beside his son quietly and reserved. When the art therapist told them that there were only five minutes left before the end of the session, Gili began to feel pressured and cried that there was not enough time to finish, that he believed that he was no good and that he ruined everything. The father sat helpless amidst the drama. At this point, the art therapist approached him and suggested that he ask Gili what he needed and how he could help him. When the father did so, at first Gili went on crying and could not answer. The father seemed to wake up and regain his composure. He began to roll a clay bounder, patted affectionately Gili's head and smiled at him. Gili calmed down gradually, described what needed to be done and they slowly started working together.

Interventions in the relationship with the art therapist. These intervention techniques typically take place when parents do not attend the parent-child art psychotherapy sessions and the art therapists must work with the student alone. Most of the time, these sessions focus on the relationship between the art therapist and the student. An attempt is made to strengthen the therapeutic alliance and the student's confidence in the art therapist. In the following example, the individual sessions with the student facilitated his return to parent-child art psychotherapy after a difficult period. Ten-year-old Ido refused to attend parent-child art psychotherapy sessions with his parents following a personal crisis after two years of joint therapy. In parental guidance, it was decided that in conjunction with the parents' discussions with him, the art therapist would ask Ido to come to an individual art therapy session to help him renew the therapeutic alliance and preserve the therapeutic space that enabled him to engage in emotional sharing. The art therapist and Ido's parents wrote him a letter which included photographs of his artworks that he produced during his two year period of parent-child art psychotherapy, as well as statements and descriptions of his emotional experiences and confused state. The conceptualization of the situation and feelings created a connection and facilitated his return to therapy with the art therapist and subsequently to parent-child art psychotherapy. This example highlights the importance of the art therapist's relationship with the client and his/her readiness to find an array of possible solutions to promote the well-being of the client.

Psycho-educational work. In the parent-child art psychotherapy model, part of the art therapist's work is also psycho-educational, such that the art therapist occasionally makes recommendations related to the world outside the art therapy room. These can include referrals for a parent to receive individual psychotherapy or a referral for couple therapy for parents who raise emotional content in sessions that is not only related to their parenthood. These may also include recommendations for specific behavioral practices at home or to encourage parents to spend more time with their children. The following example shows how the information provided to parents and specific recommendations for interventions enabled them to help their son in times of distress. Six-year-old Lior lives with his family in an area of the country which has complicated security issues. He was directed to parent-child art psychotherapy at school because of his anxiety and the trauma he experienced when a missile landed close to his home. During one of the sessions, the parents shared their concern and described that for the first time they noticed Lior shaking when the civil defense siren blared. When asked about it, he responded that he was cold. In the parental guidance sessions, the art therapist explained to his parents that this is a natural reaction to impending danger. The parents recalled situations in which they themselves had extreme physical reactions to the incoming missile sirens. The parents and art therapist engaged in shared thinking and came up with the idea of using physical activity (such as playing with a ball or jumping) to relieve and release the stress that Lior and his family felt while in the air raid shelter during an alarm.

The Systemic Setting of the Art Therapist in Parent-Child Art Psychotherapy

Many art therapists who work in parent-child art psychotherapy in the educational system are also in contact with the multidisciplinary staff who work with the student. When this relationship is optimally adapted, it can support the goals of therapy and expand the scope of work for the student. However, from time to time, as a result of disagreements between staff members, the relationship can become complex and occasionally lead to resistance on the part of the art therapist or the educational staff. Careful attention to ethical guidelines in this type of therapy is crucial, since by including the parents in the therapeutic setting, the art therapist is often exposed to confidential family information and needs to set clear boundaries for both the family members and the educational staff as to what information is passed on and what remains in the therapy room. The following example illustrates how the educational staff can help expand the circle of support for the student. Eight-year-old David was diagnosed with communication difficulties. He was referred to parent-child art psychotherapy at school to help him and his family deal with his condition. Gradually, David began to feel more understood in the sessions and for the first time in a long time he felt loved and not alone. Subsequently, at the end of the sessions his parting from his parents became problematic and dramatic. He cried, lay down on the school stairs and struggled to say goodbye to his parents when they left the art therapy room and at the school gate. At first, the educational staff found it difficult to cope with the situation and threatened to punish him. This distressed David's parents who found it difficult to trust the staff and how they were handling his pain. In response, the art therapist convened a multidisciplinary meeting to present and explain David's difficulty and how it influenced him, as well as the need for the educational staff to encourage David to engage academically after therapy or any time he did not behave appropriately at school. It was decided that David should be given time to gradually say goodbye to his parents after art therapy and be allowed to recover in a neutral space, followed by a gradual reintegration into the classroom. The discussion between the parents and staff seemed to create a feeling of trust and improved communication and after a brief period of time, David's separation from his parents at the end of art therapy improved noticeably. This case illustrates the potential for student development when various factors in the student's life work together to support growth.

The Roles of Art

Art plays a major role in parent-child art psychotherapy sessions. The role of art varies as a function of the type of session, the nature and needs of the clients at a given time and the art therapist's personality and treatment approach.

Art as a tool for emotional expression. Both the parent and the child who attend parent-child art psychotherapy use art for emotional expression. The creative process, including contact with the art materials, typically provides client and parents a sense of enjoyment, interest, and mutual and personal admiration. However, some clients perceive art as a tool to express more difficult feelings, such as distress and disappointment, which can be manifested in the creative process. Parental guidance can offer parents a space for emotional expression by observing their joint artworks with their children or by making an artwork under the guidance of the art therapist. Through this process, parents can expand their understanding of their relationships with their child. In the following example, the creative work constituted a locus for emotional expression for parent and child. Ten-year-old Shai has Attention Deficit Hyperactivity Disorder (ADHD) and difficulties understanding social situations. During parent-child art psychotherapy, both parents noticed his difficulties and struggled to perceive his creativity and other positive personality traits. In one session with his mother, the art therapist suggested that the mother and Shai make a joint drawing. Shai initially objected, but eventually they agreed to work using gouache paints. The collaborative work with his mother was moving and included expressive and joyful components. They enjoyed working together, and for the first time Shai sensed his mother's appreciation.

Expressions of connection and separation between members of the dyad through art. There are various ways in which members of the dyad can create artworks together. Depending on the goals of therapy, the art therapist can offer the parent and child a variety of possibilities for collaborative work. Work can take place simultaneously on separate platforms or jointly on one platform. Occasionally, a drawing created by one of the members of the dyad serves as a basis for the other, or both members can work together to complete an artwork. In other cases, whether initiated by the parent, child or the art therapist, the parent and child can also express themselves separately. Sometimes the initiative is individual work by each member of the dyad and at other times during the creative process, one of the members can decide to retreat from the joint work or find a separate space that accentuates his/her individuality. As a result of the joint artwork, the need for separation can be observed, as can be seen in the following example. Tomer, a nine-year-old, has Attention Deficit Disorder. He was referred to parent-child art psychotherapy at school after reports of social isolation, emotional distress and difficulties at home with his parents and a symbiotic relationship with his mother. In one of the sessions, Tomer took a small piece of paper and started working on an interesting drawing. It was evident that he was concentrating and very busy. His mother asked: "May I draw on your drawing?" Tomer did not answer her. The art therapist tried to find out whether Tomer would let his mother draw on his drawing. He apparently did not really want her to join him but found it difficult to stand up to her. When Tomer stopped momentarily, the mother assumed that he was inviting her to join him and immediately began drawing circles around his drawing. During the joint observation of the artwork, Tomer's mother commented that they had drawn an ancient war symbol, a subject that interested Tomer. Tomer was astonished and replied: "I drew a pizza." During the parental guidance sessions while observing the artwork, the parents were able to discuss the cost of Tomer's symbiotic relationship, his need for individuality and Tomer's developmental delay and deficiency for the first time.

Art functioning as a link between sessions. In each parent-child art psychotherapy session, a different dyad is present in the therapy room and art can form a bridge between the sessions. The student can choose to refer to an artwork created with the other parent or continue an artwork between sessions and as such establish a connection between sessions in which each parent was present. This occurred in the case of David (mentioned above) who used clay in therapy. In each session he chose to continue his artwork with the parent present in the art therapy room, as though not differentiating which parent was there. In the parental guidance sessions, the parents stated that they were experiencing marital difficulties and often argued and were angry at each other at home and had trouble communicating. The parents stated that at home during their arguments as well as in therapy, David was trying to bring his parents together again and generate continuity between them through artwork. The parents' understanding of the situation enabled them to open up and talk to David about the situation at home. Occasionally, as in this example, the links between the therapy sessions are established during the parental guidance sessions where the parents and art therapist observe the artworks together and can follow what occurred in the sessions when they were not present.

Art as a space for reflection. The joint sessions between the parent and the child incorporate participation in creative processes, but also involve the observation and reflection of the process and art product. The observation of the artworks provides a basis for a discussion, the expression of thoughts and emotions, and is a means to weigh in on the feelings that accompany the creative process. Subsequently, in the parental guidance sessions there is an opportunity to review and observe the artworks while expanding the parents' observational skills during the year. The following example illustrates this process with Gal, a three and a half year old who was referred to parent-child art psychotherapy in his kindergarten because of fears that arose after a dangerous security situation in the area where he lives. Gal was confused about the need to stay in the air raid shelter and the noise of missile sirens and gun fire. During a session with his mother (who had suffered from childhood trauma), she wanted to make a pretty drawing, and throughout the creative process, she held Gal's hand with the paintbrush, guided his hand and painted for him. In some areas of the page she painted alone and at the end of the process, she wrote Gal's name on the artwork and even praised him for the beauty of the work. During a session with his father, he preferred to have

Gal create something alone. He remained to the side and admired all the mixing, marks and splashes of color. In parental guidance, the art therapist placed the two artworks in front of the parents. The paintings reflected the parents' different ways of dealing with Gal, one from a place of total control (the mother) and the other from a place of freedom and admiration without reciprocity or closeness (the father). Gaining this understanding allowed each parent to learn from the other parent what behavior was least present in his/her interactions with Gal and to generate some flexibility in their approach while changing their relationship and communication with Gal. This example illustrates the differences that can be associated with each parent and the extent to which parent-child art psychotherapy can help broaden the observation of their parenthood and its meaning.

The Emotional Content That Emerges in the Parent-Child Art Psychotherapy Process

The parent-child art psychotherapy work format encourages work on emotional content that would probably not be dealt with in art therapy sessions in the education system. The parent-child relationship and more generally extended family relationships constitute the core of this work. These relationships affect the student's behavior considerably. At times other content can be elicited in the sessions that deal with aggression. During parent-child art psychotherapy sessions, the clients can work with and regulate aggression and in other cases, aggression is given a space for expression and meaning within the context of the relationship. Finally, additional content focuses on the clients including their condition and functioning, as well as coping skills and challenges in their lives. This was the case for Nili, a three and a half year old in kindergarten who was referred to parent-child art psychotherapy based on the kindergarten teacher's reports of restlessness and pressure during a dramatic play. During the intake sessions, Nili's parents did not know how to attribute her difficulties to events in her life. When asked about their family and major events in their lives, they mentioned that when Nili was about one year old, her older sister was very ill and as a result her parents were away from home for approximately one month, during which time Nili's grandparents looked after her. The parents assumed that Nili would not remember this period and that her behavior had nothing to do with the family event. During one session with her father, Nili chose to use medical equipment and began examining her father. She indicated precisely those symptoms that her sister suffered from during her illness. During parental guidance, a reflective discussion about the joint game was held and the father told the mother that he was now confident that Nili's difficulties were related to the "abandonment" that she had experienced and her trauma in having to be separated from her parents during her sister's illness. With the help of the art therapist, the parents gradually understood that it was important to talk to Nili in an age-appropriate way about the "secret" and in this way release her from her unspoken memories of the incident that occurred in her infancy.

Summary and Conclusion

This chapter addressed parent-child art psychotherapy within the educational system. The sections outlined a dedicated working model illustrated with examples from the field. The decision on the part of the educational system to incorporate parents into the students' art therapy process is grounded in the firm belief that this is the most appropriate way of improving the functioning of a particular student within the system. This is carried out by observing the family setting and specifically by focusing on improving the parent-child relationship. Since students are in school when most parents are at work, the decision to engage in this type of therapy within the educational system requires a great deal of thought and planning in terms of the treatment schedule and conducting individual therapy sessions without the parents when they cannot participate in a session. This challenge highlights the need for dedication, flexibility and motivation on the part of all parties to successfully uphold the therapy setting and benefit from the therapeutic process. The core of the parent-child art psychotherapy session is the creative work through which the relationship between the parent and the child is reflected, and by which processes of change can be promoted. Sometimes, these processes can help establish a closer relationship between the parent and child through collaborative creative work whereas at other times the artwork promotes separation that is age-appropriate to the student by working on separate art formats. The role of art in the therapeutic process is diverse and varies as a function of the type of session and the nature and needs of the clients at a given time, in addition to the art therapist's personality and therapeutic approach. The art therapist guides the process and helps to forge the relationship between the student, his/her parents and the educational system.

References

Ben-Aaron, M., Harel, J., Kaplan, H., & Patt, R. (2001). *Mother–child and father–child psychotherapy: A manual for the treatment of relational disturbances in childhood*. London: Whurr Publishers.

Bowlby, J. (1979). *The making and breaking of affection al bonds*. London: Tavistock.

Dancette-De Bresson (2016). *Dyad art therapy: Birth of modality. A research paper in the department of creative arts therapies*. Partial fulfillment for the degree of Master of Arts. Montreal: Concordia University.

Fonagy, P., Gergely, G., & Target, M. (2007). The parent–infant dyad and the construction of the subjective self. *Journal of Child Psychology and Psychiatry*, *48*(3/4), 288–328.

Fraiberg, S., Adelson, E., & Shapiro, V. (1975). Ghosts in the nursery: Psychoanalytic approach to the problems of impaired infant-mother relationship. *Journal of the American Academy of Child Psychiatry*, *14*, 387–421.

Gavron, T. (2013). Meeting on common ground: Assessing parent–child relationships through the joint painting procedure. *Art Therapy: Journal of the American Art Therapy Association*, *30*(1), 12–19.

Gavron, T. (2017). The joint painting procedure: Parents and children creating shared space. *Art Therapy Online*, *8* (1).

Harel, J., Kaplan, H., Avimeir-Patt, R., Ben-Aaron, M. (2006). The child's active role in mother-child, father-child psychotherapy: A psychodynamic approach to the treatment of relational disturbances. *Psychology and Psychotherapy: Theory, Research and Practice*, 79(1), 23–36.

Kaplan, H., Harel, Y., & Avimeir-Patt, R. (2010). *Parent-child psychotherapy, a meeting place between the therapeutic practice and theory*. Haifa: University of Haifa, Department of Psychology (in Hebrew).

Kyung, S.K., Choi, S.N., & Park, S.W. (2016). A narrative inquiry into a mother- child art therapy experience: A self- exploration of the therapist and the mother. *The Arts in Psychotherapy*, *47*, 23–30.

Mahler, M.S., Pine, F., & Bergman, A. (1975). *The psychological birth of the human infant*. New York: Basic Books.

Markman Zinemanas, D. (1994). A description of the art therapy intervention model for parent-child groups, for children with drawing impairments. *Art Therapy*, *3*, 50–35 (in Hebrew).

Meyerowitz-Kats, J., & Reddick, D. (2017). *Art therapy in early years*. New York: Routledge.

Minuchin, S. (2007). *Forty years of family therapy*. Lecture at the meeting of the Israel Association for Family and Couple Therapy. Ramat Efal (in Hebrew).

Proulx, L. (2003). *Strengthening emotional ties through parent-child dyad art therapy*. London: Jessica Kingsley publishers.

Prooulx, L. (2017). *Attachment informed art therapy: Strengthening emotional ties throughout the lifetime*. Lucille Proulx.

Regev, D., & Snir, S. (2014). Working with parents in parent-child art psychotherapy. *The Arts in Psychotherapy*, *41*, 511–518.

Regev, D., & Snir, S. (2015). Objectives, interventions and challenges in parent-child art psychotherapy. *The Arts in Psychotherapy*, *42*, 50–56.

Regev, D., & Snir, S. (2017). *Parent-child art psychotherapy*. New York: Routledge.

Shapira, G. (2018). Moving together – the parent-child art psychotherapy approach in the education system. In S. Snir & D. Regev (Eds.), *When arts therapy meets the education system in Israel: Applied aspects*. The Emili Sagol Research Center: University of Haifa (in Hebrew).

Stern, D.N. (1995). *The motherhood constellation: A unified view of parent-infant psychotherapy*. New-York: Basic Books.

Stern, D.N. (1998). Mothers' emotional needs. *Pediatrics*, *102*(Supplement E1), 1250–1252.

Tamir, R., & Regev, D. (2020). Characteristics of parent-child art psychotherapy in the education system. *The Arts in Psychotherapy*, 101725.

Taylor Buck, E., Dent-Brown, K., & Parry, G. (2013). Exploring a dyadic approach to art psychotherapy with children and young people: A survey of British art psychotherapists. *International Journal of Art Therapy: Formerly Inscape*, *18*(1), 20–28.

Winnicott, D.W. (1971). *Playing and reality*. Middlesex: Penguin.

7 The "Open Studio" Model in Educational Frameworks

Anat Heller

Introduction

The education system today is confronted with numerous challenges related to its efforts to provide an optimal educational experience for all. These issues are impacted by the rapid pace of progress in technology, efforts to adapt programs to modern needs, and also the difficulties involved in creating diverse programs to respond to the needs of the younger more realistic generation attuned to self-development and the accelerated pace of life. School curricula tend to emphasize mathematics, sciences and foreign languages. In contrast, expressive and emotional language is neither directly addressed nor a core subject in many schools. As a result, there is a widening disparity between cognition-oriented technological orientations and students' ability to develop their emotional intelligence, which can lead to isolation and problems coping with emotional situations.

This chapter presents a therapeutic model named the "Open Studio," which is designed to contribute to narrowing the gap between cognition and emotion, and between physicality and social conduct, to create a complete and holistic form of self-expression. Section one presents the "Open Studio" concept, its theoretical foundation, its guiding therapeutic principles and describes a structured Open Studio model called "Bridge to Connection" that was implemented for a group of primary school students. The second section reviews a study on an Open Studio in a primary school and focuses on the contribution of the model to developing emotional coping skills and in particular reflective skills and tools to enhance self-efficacy.

The "Open Studio" is an approach in the field of art therapy that views clients as creators and artists who enter a space that allows them to experience processes of expression and creation with materials (Block, Harris, & Laing, 2005; McNiff, 2000). The Open Studio is a space that makes diverse creative materials available from raw to recycled materials, utensils and work tools. The word "open" affixed to "studio" relates to the essence of this approach that allows clients to experience an openness to a flow of ideas and freedom of choice in the studio at different stages of the process. Participation in an Open Studio is voluntary, and the themes in the artistic process are chosen by the client. Similarly, the work process, choice of materials and mode of expression are not determined by the art therapist. Clients are invited to learn from their experiences while making progress in their work, accompanied by the art therapist. The length of time working and breaks are determined by the clients, as are decisions regarding the fate of art products. Art therapists encourage clients to keep their artworks in the studio to allow for a learning process, and at the end of each period the clients decide which pieces of artwork to recycle, give to someone or throw away. All these decisions are made by the clients.

Although a number of clients work in an Open Studio at the same time, work is individual. Unlike group work, where a common therapeutic goal is central to therapy, in an Open Studio the therapeutic goal is likely to be personal and vary from client to client. Clients evolve in an Open Studio in relation to their personal goals and as guided by their own needs and desires. Choices regarding the creative work are made by being attuned to personal wishes in the "here and now" and accurately reflect the needs of each client separately in real time. Because of the nature of this work, an Open Studio is defined as individual art therapy in the presence of a group. Clients in an Open Studio learn to distance themselves from their environment and to manage their needs and emotions in relation to themselves and their environment.

Art therapists in an Open Studio accompany clients throughout the creative process and their personal choices and provide artistic guidance according to need. One of the key roles of art therapists is to mediate creative processes to promote participants' learning about themselves. Art therapists employ phenomenological explorative discourse to help clients develop reflective skills. One of the ways of mediating this is through modeling, where art therapists create in the presence of clients. They do not only "explain" but also "dos" while employing a range of techniques, materials and new adaptations. Art therapists can consult the creators around them openly about their work and in this way provide a special experience of learning and an eye-level relationship. They are responsible for the work time framework which is set according to needs and restrictions.

Theoretical Background

The Open Studio concept is based on a number of theoretical approaches, each of which, in its own way, contributes to constructing the Open Studio's approach and implementation. The key approach is "art as therapy" (Hyland Moon, 2002; Kramer, 2001; McNiff, 2000). This approach sees the healing power of art in people's natural need for play, activity and expression. The language of art is the language of materials and is perceived by the senses, thus enabling personal and interpersonal expression and communication, especially when using words is difficult. Engaging in creative activities enables the expression and release of troubling and chaotic emotions and repositions them in esthetic structures within the frames of language and art (Betensky, 1995; Hazut, 2014; McNiff, 2000). Hazut (2014) noted that artistic expression that bypasses internal censorship can foster creativity, complex thinking and flexibility, and as such contributes to changes in perceptions of self-esteem and self-confidence.

Another key Open Studio approach is the phenomenological approach, which explores a phenomenon (from the Greek *phaenesthai*). Its modern beginnings date back to the turn of the 20th century where it emerged as a philosophical reaction to empiricism that strove for absolute truth within the objectivity of science. Husserl and his student Heidegger were among those who developed phenomenological philosophy. They argued that true reality was and will always be something unknown, impossible to examine that must be considered a subjective event (Heidegger, 1927; Husserl, 1967). Phenomenology is important as a methodology in research as a means of collecting qualitative information about the artistic and creative work process (Moustakas, 1994).

In the therapeutic language, phenomenology refers to observing and describing through the senses, emotions, dreams, memories, fantasies and everything passing through the brain or personal consciousness and belongs to the field of mental experiences (Betensky, 1995). Phenomenology, because it deals with the age-old dilemma of the connection between external "objective" reality and emotions and personal thoughts, allows clients to return to subjectivity, to the experience as perceived by the client, in terms of the self. This can increase clients' understanding of themselves and their environment (Betensky, 1977). In art therapy, phenomenology involves reflective discourse. This is how clients and art therapists describe their processes and visual creations. They are encouraged to do so by postponing interpretation and suspending criticism or judgment (Betensky, 1977). The subjective observer's position is the pillar of the Open Studio and enables clients to observe themselves and their unique expressions. It also involves a grasp of the relationship between a seen thing as a phenomenon and its perception. Phenomenological observation deploys diverse qualities of clients' artworks and is likely to also be part of follow-up and assessment in the therapeutic process.

Another approach influencing work in the Open Studio is the "Experiential Learning" approach to learning (Kolb, 2014). Dewey (1938) was one of the first to point to the association between learning and personal experience. He argued that not every experience will lead to learning, but that for learning to occur, there must be a reflective process of thinking about the experience and structuring it in consciousness. In Experiential Learning, knowledge acquired in one area can be transferred to others. Similarly, emotional and cognitive knowledge acquired through experiences in the Open Studio can be applied to other areas of life (Bandura, 1989). The concept of Experiential Learning comes from the field of education, which exists in the studio and applies to personal and emotional contents. This connects the educational and therapeutic frameworks. This interface is important because the education system and art therapists both tend to separate education from therapy and emphasize their differences. Schools may thus be more accepting of a therapeutic approach that implements familiar concepts.

Two other crucial concepts associated with work in the Open Studio are reflection and the experience of self-efficacy. These concepts emerge from studio work (Heller, 2015) and are examined in the second section of this chapter. “Reflection is an important human activity in which people recapture their experience, think about it, mull it over and evaluate it” (Boud and Walker, 1985. p. 19). As art therapists, we encourage our clients to recreate processes, observe them, explore what was discovered and produce new understandings. Learning and new insights can affect life as part of the healing process. The ability to reflect is intrinsically related to the associative nature of thinking (Boud, Keogh, & Walker, 2013). A meaningful piece of information is absorbed by the observer and associated with another piece of information in the individual’s internal world. Metaphorically, this produces a type of cluster of unique personal knowledge. The work in an Open Studio and the reflection on it build a network of experiences based on what happened in the studio and links to other events and occurrences in each participant’s internal and external worlds. This expanded experience then acquires a structure and can be parsed. This component is extremely important because it responds to the query of whether what occurs in the Open Studio carries over to the outside world. Art therapy in a school framework makes reflection within the studio even more important because in academic settings as well, reflection plays a central role in thinking and understanding. Reflective thinking requires learners to conceptualize learning and invites behavioral change (Boud et al., 2013a; Dewey 1933). However, despite the importance of reflective thinking, schools do not sufficiently emphasize on learning reflective language as a skill that can foster learning and expressive processes (Moon, 2013; Zohar, 2004).

The reflective process in the studio takes place at all stages and in diverse forms. There are different types of reflection (Schön, 1983). Reflection occurs in action, for example, at the intentionality stage before starting to create. The action involves choosing representations describing the self to awaken self-awareness. Reflection characterizes choices students make and what they mean to them. Another example of reflection in action is found in the creative process when students encounter a problem or hurdle, where they must describe the sequence of events to overcome it; in other words, they need to reflect in a way they can understand and then decide what to do. Another type of reflection is reflection on action in the last stage of the studio, the observation stage. The creative process has ended, and the students look back and describe the steps taken. At this stage, thinking assembles the sequence, the problems and how they coped with them. Reflection allows the rational outcomes of work to remain in one's consciousness in a structured and organized manner.

The other key concept linked to Open Studio work is experiencing "self-efficacy." The concept of self-efficacy derives from Bandura's Social Learning theory and is defined as the extent of people's belief in their ability to influence events in their lives (Bandura, 1989). The concept self-efficacy refers to people's judgment of their own abilities to organize or carry out behavior or a series of behaviors successfully to achieve a desired outcome. The concept differentiates between existing skills, belief in one's own abilities and recognizing the results of actions (Bandura, 1986). Peer groups are the main agents for developing and validating self-efficacy. A low sense of social self-efficacy is likely to impede the formation of positive social relationships (Bandura, 1997). Students in the studio who are part of a peer group have opportunities to experience their self-efficacy and develop it in creative processes, reflective thinking, through interactions with other students, mediated by their significant adults.

Description of the Working Model

There are various Open Studio models. This chapter focuses on the structured "Bridge to Connection" model inspired by the Open Studio operating in an adult psychiatric day ward at the Ziv Medical Center in Safed, Israel. This model was developed and has been studied over the years through collaboration with art therapists, students and professionals who work there as well as the clients themselves. The model is characterized by fixed stages the clients go through in the studio, of which creation in art materials is one part. This model served as the basis for developing my Open Studio model in the school setting.

"Bridge to Connection" Model in the Educational Framework

In 2011, I was employed by the Open Studio at the Ziv Medical Center and in supervising art therapists for the Ministry of Education. I realized that in both places there was a need to find additional ways of expressing thoughts and emotions, overcoming self-expression and interpersonal communication difficulties, developing a motivation for investigation, and nurturing independence and responsibility. In both settings, there was a high demand for art therapy for a large number of clients but few allocated therapy hours or art therapists. Frameworks having to deal with these issues usually turn to group therapies. In this situation, individual clients' needs are only treated to the extent that they correspond to the needs of the group. This can also create therapist burnout, and detachment from the joy and vitality of creativity.

Many clients in schools are referred by teachers or school counselors to art therapy for difficulties related to self-expression: "The student does not participate in class or the student never stops talking, he/she has potential, but never uses it, he/she is socially withdrawn, struggles to explain him/herself" or "he/she refuses to take responsibility for doing what he/she is asked to do," "he/she has no motivation." This makes it difficult to define a therapeutic framework that can support a student or define a therapeutic goal to respond to these difficulties. The uniqueness of an Open Studio lies in its flexibility and ability to permit diverse emphases and goals. It is flexible in terms of its characteristics and the number of participants and is multidimensional in terms of the depth of artistic work as therapy and the way people learn about themselves. For all these reasons, it made sense to set up an Open Studio within the school space.

Goals. The goals of an in-school Open Studio emanate from the therapeutic goals of the clients. The studio's ability to relate to individuals in a group framework allows for the delineation of a wide range of therapeutic emotional, cognitive, functional, social, learning, developmental resilience resource goals (Heller, 2015). For example, a student who has problems expressing emotions and for whom the therapeutic goal is to develop expressive ability can be placed in the same group as a student who feels socially rejected for whom the therapeutic goal is self-empowerment and strengthening of self-image and self-efficacy.

Target population. Students who receive therapy in an Open Studio do not need prior knowledge of art or artistic abilities. However, students with needs linked to high levels of dependency or regulation are likely to struggle with this type of independent work such that the ratio of art therapists to clients needs to be increased in this case.

Advantages. The advantages of art therapy in an Open Studio in a school framework are also related more generally to the issues of art therapy in an educational framework:

- Difficulty allocating therapy hours in the light of students' many needs. In an Open Studio, work with numerous students is feasible, so that more students' needs are personally addressed.
- Heterogeneity in students' ages and developmental stages, sometimes from the same class, make group creation and determining a uniform therapeutic goal difficult. In an Open Studio, individual therapeutic goals can be maintained while still working in the presence of a group.
- School systems are typically characterized by the need to see each student's uniqueness, and not enough human resources to do so. In the studio, each student gets an opportunity to present his/her artwork and inner world.
- Since the success of art therapy is linked to a systemic vision, when a studio operates within a school it constitutes a link between the student and the school system. There is separation from and integration with the educational framework, and a blurring and minimizing of the social stigma of art therapy. Clients coming as creators do not have to

cope with the stigma of difference or disability. Typically, as soon as students understand what an Open Studio is, other students want to join the program.

- A studio, in its essence, allows for the development of learning skills such as phenomenological language, thus enabling communication and expressive skills.
- An approach that sees every student as an artist in a studio, who can carry out independent work and is directed to take responsibility and initiative, contribute to strengthening self-esteem, motivation to act and self-efficacy.

Cooperation. To develop a functional model for a school framework, ideas, studio stages and students' needs all have to be researched, understood and operationalized. Part of this involves structuring a program consistent with the school framework. To achieve cohesion between therapy and class and to generate cooperation, the program should first be presented to the principal, counselors, teachers and other administrative personnel. Without their approval, cooperation and enthusiasm, it is impossible to engage in this type of program in schools.

Therapeutic Setting

An in-studio session lasts approximately one and a half hours, or two class periods. It takes place once a week in a place defined as the studio space. This can be the school's art room (coordinated with art teachers) or another designated room. Sometimes the Open Studio space is a classroom space, where the art materials and mobile work boards are wheeled into the room on a trolley each time there is a session. Each session has a fixed-stage work framework.

"Bridge to Connection" model stages. Studio sessions begin with a short discussion constituting the transitional text describing the shift from classroom to group, connection and intimacy. This is followed by four fixed, consistent stages in each session:

First stage – physical warmup. The purpose of this stage is to get the body ready to act, to create self-awareness of the inner-body, mind and emotional processes. This is done in a group in a playful manner and includes breathing exercises, games with accessories such as a ball, balloons, hoops and the like.

Second stage – intentionality. The purpose of this stage is to instill and practice metaphorical language to describe an internal experience. Since most of the students struggle to describe their feelings in depth, we use objects (cards, small-world images, materials from nature, journals, etc.) that can be projected and esthetically distanced from the subject that is often too difficult to articulate. A new object is chosen each time as a "here and now" experience representing a student's experience concretely (seen externally) and metaphorically (seen internally). This stage ends when the art therapist inquires what each student intends to do through art: unload emotions, express him/herself, explore materials or a topic.

Third stage – creative stage. Here students approach the "materials buffet." Some are always available such as materials and utensils as well as office equipment and work surfaces. As a studio progresses, more and more materials are added. The students can act independently but can also consult the art therapist.

Fourth stage – observation. The purpose of this stage is a collective reflection to build awareness. The students learn to observe a phenomenon – their own and others' artwork – without judgment or criticism. Artworks are placed in front of the group and each student in turn describes the process he/she underwent. The other students constitute an attentive audience, asking phenomenological, non-interpretive questions such that the presenter's awareness of him/herself and his/her abilities can be structured. Repetition and consistency produce consciousness and confidence within the fixed stages, whereas the creative processes and content change all the time.

Assessment of the work and therapy process takes place on two levels. The first consists of personally observing a number of artworks. Students who have already learned the principles of phenomenological inquiry define their artistic style together with the art therapist and can make decisions about the creative stages in terms of a work topic or its re-organization. The second level is a broader personal exhibition, which is best carried out after several works have accumulated. Setting up the exhibition requires all artworks to be spread out, categorized and the internal and external perspectives delineated. From the students' point of view, this is an exercise involving choice, making decisions and esthetically arranging materials and topics that are of interest to them. From the point of view of the art therapist, this is an opportunity to view the process through the phenomenology of the art sequence, examine the students' development according to their therapeutic goals and assess their progress. The exhibition comes at the end of the process of preparing and getting to know themselves. Esthetic arrangement and a familiar audience – the group of students – strengthens the experience and validates the achievements of the entire process. Note that this is an internal exhibition not directed at an audience.

Work rules. An Open Studio invites contact with the internal world. Thus, rules supporting the process of turning the studio into a "safe place" need to be defined. These rules, which form a "participation contract," are stated clearly at the start of the Open Studio program and are part of the therapeutic contract.

Participants respect one another, the materials and the artwork. This type of discourse allows art therapists to intervene when there are displays of aggression or disrespect among students or directed towards themselves. Respecting the art materials means taking responsibility for all the studio resources and how they are used. Artworks constitute the process. This is because sketches, experiments or products of ongoing processes are evidence and milestones of development that should be treated with respect.

Studio work takes place without judgment or criticism. At a personal level, the creative process confronts students with the disparity between fantasy and the real world. Not once does this gap represent experiences of frustration and anger. Hence, the journey to judgment and criticism is very short. At a group level, there can be tensions and comparisons between students. The need to be accepted, fall in line or stand out often occurs when students belittle their peers judgmentally or critically. For this reason, studio art therapists need to immediately stop and address any judgmental or critical comments, propose alternative references and explain the impact of this discourse. This rule emphasizes coping and correct conduct and is a guarantor of a safe place for expression.

Do not "plant ideas" in others. When students create and expose their artworks to others, there is a tendency in the "audience" to react interpretively from within their own conceptual world. This interpretation is likely to bias and affect self-expression and/or conceptualize a topic/idea the art maker did not have in mind or was not yet ready to address. Therefore, students learn mainly to ask questions rather than put forward their opinions or interpretations. This type of interest serves inquiry learning and phenomenological observation and allows the process to take place at an appropriate time and place.

Maintaining confidentiality and privacy of group participants. This rule defines the studio as a safe place, sets boundaries and strengthens the role of a studio as a container. This occurs when both art therapists and clients keep the content that emerges in the studio confidential and do not disclose them to others, students or staff outside the studio.

These rules constitute guidelines for the students and help them conduct themselves in the studio space where their experiences are less restricted and freer than in the educational framework. For art therapists, the rules serve to signpost the therapeutic space and as an anchor for conduct within boundaries and behavior in this space. If a student deviates from the rules, the art therapist immediately draws the student's attention to the violation and points out that studio participation is his or her choice and obligates them to obey these rules. In my experience, no student confronted with the rules has ever chosen to leave the studio.

Clinical Example

For a more vivid depiction of how an Open Studio experience unfolds, imagine a film about a group of four boys, Nir, Gilad, Yaron and Noam, all 5th graders. We will join Noam, who describes a studio session, and attempt to understand through his eyes how it appears. Text is inspired by conversations with 5th graders, who participated in the school Open Studio, and relates to the first few weeks of its operation (Heller, 2015).

> Wednesday, first and second lessons, we have an Open Studio. We all got to the studio when the bell rang (actually the school's art room, now the studio room). Dana (art therapist) asked us to sit in a circle. She gave Nir a card labelled "opening circle" and Nir read from it: "I the artist think about myself and choose to share something with group members." Everybody could say whatever he or she wanted. I talked about a trip I took to visit my uncles in Ashdod. When everyone finished, I asked Dana to read the second card: "physical warmup": "I the artist connect to my body and senses and prepare them for creative work." Today we played a movement game when each person invented a movement and the others repeated it. It was a little like the game "Copycat," but without moving from the circle. Then we did the opposite movement. At the end we took slow deep breaths. Dana explained that this was associated with the body and breathing control and that it was good for all sorts of situations. Yaron read from the card "intentionality": "I the artist look at things on the table and look for the 'thing' that connects me the most to what I am sensing and feeling now. Then I can choose and direct myself in studio work." We sat around the table. Dana took out a lot of plastic animal figures (like those we had as small children) out of a box. She asked each one of us to pay attention to what was happening in each of us now, what our mood was and then decide which animals represented us at the moment or which animal we felt a connection with. I immediately connected to the tiger. Today we were also handed a page with a list of emotions. Dana asked us to look at our animal and see which emotion we connected to. When my turn came, I talked about the tiger...sometimes I dream about one. They are very frightening animals. Dana asked me questions about the tiger I was holding in my hand: about his color, what material he was made of, what I could say about his movement, what drew my attention. Then she asked me to imagine who this tiger was, how old he was and what he liked to do. In the list of emotions, bored is what corresponded to me best. Then she asked me what I wanted to do with boredom today, to express it in art? Or perhaps to put boredom aside and focus on something else? I chose to put it aside and to continue building the robot from the last time.
>
> After everyone had done intentionality, Gilad did not want to read, so Nir read the card about art making: "I the artist give myself the freedom to create with diverse materials in the studio, without knowing in advance where it will lead." Everyone began to work. Dana took colored paper and began to staple them together. I worked on the robot and did not know how to attach the hands. Dana suggested a number

> of possibilities for gluing them and taught me how to use each type of glue, and when. In the end I chose hot glue. The time passed quickly, and we only had 20 minutes left. Dana stopped us even though I really wanted to go on for a little while longer. We sat in front of the art works in a semi-circle. Both Yaron and I wanted to read out loud. Dana told us to work it out between us. Yaron let me do it. "Observation": "I the artist observe the process I have undergone: starting with what I felt at the start and warmup, via my choice of an object that would represent me in the intentionality, working with the materials, to producing art; my personal journey today." When my turn came, I stood and explained how I had made the robot and what I had added today. Dana asked me how I had started the day, she reminded me that I had chosen a tiger and what happened to my boredom. I said I had fun and that making a robot made me happy. My friends asked me questions: How did I put the robot together, what was hardest and also why I had made the robot a boy. When Dana heard this, she jumped up and said that this was interpretation and we do not interpret but can only ask the presenter to elaborate on the artwork. Yaron changed the question and asked whether the robot had a gender. I said it was clear it was a boy. I used to be shy about speaking in front of everyone, but now I am really okay with it.

This description shows the flow between the different segments and how the tiger figure Noam connected to at the beginning developed into an entire experience. From my experience, learning phenomenological, descriptive language helps students develop metaphoric language and expands their ability to express experiences themselves. Noam expressed his fear metaphorically using the tiger, he stayed with his fear when talking about the tiger's features, but when he was asked directly what he felt, he chose the word boredom, in other words, he chose not to relate to his fears directly. The art therapist allowed him to choose how to manage his "boredom" and he chose to set it aside and be with his stronger points of building a robot.

Employing didactic accessories such as tables, posters or emotion cards create a bank of concepts which are learned and expanded. In this example, the cards written by the art therapist Galit Oren conceptualize the transition from stage to stage and are an auxiliary tool for students that helps them concentrate and internalize the role of the stages that are not related to active creation. Sometimes, there is resistance to these stages (physical warmup, intentionality and observation). In my view, it would be wrong to decide to eliminate them since each has therapeutic importance which can be explained to the participants. In the creative stage, the art therapist continues the mediating work. The participants' experiences and investigations are the building blocks to greater self-efficacy. In observation, there is a phenomenological reflection. When students present their artwork and this presentation is combined with questions, this can help re-organize the experience into a distinct structure that becomes part of consciousness.

This vignette described the relationship between students. Sometimes, there are moments of tension or conflict. In most cases, the art therapist will stop, focus on the difficulty, and clarify how in the students' opinion artists try to solve problems, such as an absence of ideas, being stuck, copying, "stealing ideas," the lack of materials, etc. The art space provides answers to many professional questions in the creative process, as well as a place to resolve difficulties in the emotional, interpersonal and social space.

Thus overall, the structured Open Studio model "Bridge to Connection" at school provides a clear and defined framework for changing content from students' internal and external worlds. It is a place where the language of art, the language of description, and the metaphoric, abstract language for physical, emotional and cognitive expression are learned while working with materials. Students learn how to observe these features and control themselves emotionally.

The connection between the therapeutic space and the educational space within the Open Studio framework is a natural one. In the studio, things are learned experientially, and kindle curiosity and the motivation to investigate. Providing an Open Studio in school legitimizes the importance of the emotional and cognitive parts of the self. Sometimes there are conflicts between the system's needs (school events for example) and therapeutic needs (maintaining a regular therapeutic routine). Some teachers view the studio as a place that rewards students, so that if they misbehave in class, they are not allowed to go to the studio. Another difficulty occurs when the staff fail to understand that the therapeutic space is a closed space. On occasion, they enter the studio space, which is experienced as intrusive and disrespectful to the therapeutic framework. This can be prevented proactively by informing the staff about the nature of the studio and how therapy unfolds in this space.

The flexibility of an Open Studio serves various purposes and can thus respond to the needs of a variety of students. Once students become familiarized with the concept and become more independent, more students can participate at one time. The Open Studio model has various levels and components, each of which call for profound inquiry. The second section of this chapter presents a study I conducted on the impact of the Open Studio on developing students' reflective ability and self-efficacy.

Study of an Open Studio in a Primary School

Open Studio is a field with many layers, each of which can be studied more profoundly. The study I conducted as part of my doctoral work had two main goals: (1) to examine the contribution of work in the studio to the development of students' reflective abilities and specifically which conditions enabled reflection and the performance quality of verbal descriptions when working in the studio; (2) to clarify whether participation in an Open Studio affected self-efficacy. Since experiencing self-efficacy is a significant factor in experiencing success and the motivation to develop, I examined which components of self-efficacy are present in the Open Studio environment and how the work in the studio affects it.

The sample was composed of eight boys and eight girls aged 11–12, who were all 5th grade students enrolled in regular education. These students were placed in four groups, two groups of girls and two groups of boys. Students were chosen for the program by the school counselor and homeroom teacher based on issues related to self-expression in class, introversion, problems establishing social relationships, self-regulation problems or middling academic proficiency. The students were informed that they had the right to take part in the studio but were not obligated to do so. The program was made up of 20 sessions led by art therapists, where each group worked in the studio for a double period (90 minutes).

Reflective process. To examine the reflective process, conversations with students in the intentionality and observation processes were documented. Further reflections were obtained from semi-structured interviews conducted at the end of the process. A qualitative analysis of the texts revealed that reflection could be classified categories related to carrying out reflection, organizing content and expression during art therapy, the art therapist's work and qualities of reflective ability.

Carrying out reflection. For reflection to occur, the individual must focus on it, identify it as a goal and allocate time and place. The findings revealed that physically, just sitting in a place where reflective discourse occurs contributed to listening and focusing. Emotionally, the location contributed to the strength of self-importance experiences. Sitting in a semi-circle with one student in the center presenting his/her process and artwork is reminiscent of an actor surrounded by an encouraging audience that sometimes claps when a presentation ends. Some students even bowed spontaneously at the end of a performance. In terms of time, there is continual tension in the Open Studio between students' desire to create freely and the art therapist's will to structure the process. The findings showed that reflection did not occur spontaneously and that art therapists had to be assertive for it to happen at all.

Another component involved in carrying out reflection is the language through which processes and their outcomes are described. In the program itself, phenomenological language was used, which by nature deals with describing and examining phenomena objectively, subjectively and the relationship between them. Anyone who has learned a new language knows there are obstacles exposing users to difficulties, and even mockery. The findings revealed that memorizing the studio's rules contributed to creating an atmosphere of respect and reduced the level of judgment and criticism. At the same time, acquiring a descriptive-phenomenological language contributed to better reflection.

Organizing content and expression. Analysis of sequences of reflection revealed that when reflection took place at a number of points on the process continuum, both within and at the end, information on the topic concerning the students could be gathered. For example, a student said in his opening text that his uncle had a horse, thus mentioning his own experiences. Later, in the physical warmup led by the art therapist he referred to imaginary lines in the space (he made movements of straight, crooked lines and the like). During intentionality, he chose a horse which he described concretely (structure, material, color on the horse's body). In this discussion the art therapist invited him to tap his internal experience about the horse which triggered metaphorical speech (the horse gallops like a storm) as well as imaginary speech (the horse belongs to a king). In the creative process, the boy copied a drawing of expressionistic horses. In the final stage of observation, the student could, through reflection, see most of the process dimensions, materials, action and the meaning he ascribed to his work and categorize it as a complete unit.

Art therapists' work. The qualitative analysis of reflections demonstrated the contribution of the art therapists' mediation to the descriptive qualities of the students' speech. Employing phenomenological questions broadened the range of description of an object from a concrete description to one that integrates metaphorical abstract thinking: "What can you say about choice of materials? What can you say about the range of colors? What draws your eye? What would this image want to do now? Where is it at this moment? What is special about it?" Another interesting finding showed that students learned to mediate through other students' questions.

Quality of reflective ability. The findings showed a change in two components of reflective ability. The first relates to the quality of reflection. This was measured using Bain's et al. (1999) five level scale of reflective quality. This model divides descriptive quality hierarchically into five categories: reporting, responding, relating, reasoning and reconstructing. At the start of work in the studio, most students evidenced the first three levels of reporting, responding and relating. For example: "I chose a bird man. I copied his wings and made a shield....I wrote my name, and then I added colors." Towards the end of the work in the studio, the students successfully developed a higher level of descriptive language that included reasoning and reconstructing. For example:

> I can choose my life the way I want. If I decide I want to have a painful life, I can choose the color red. If I want a good life, like yellow, which glows, then I will have a good life. I have to choose the way.

The second component relates to how reflective discourse is described with reference to the "objective" and "subjective" points of view. "Objective" descriptions relate, phenomenologically, to the physical and concrete qualities of the materials, the processes as perceived by the senses and for which there is collective agreement (color, shape, size, texture, etc.). For example: "The swan is transparent, small and rough. It has round lines and a splash." The "Subjective" descriptions relate to the qualities of the object or process reflected from the inner world. Here, more projective, emotional and imaginary expressions are voiced. For example: "The material was pleasant and sometimes cold...it is like the color white is that lonely. Connected to loneliness...there are things that I am tired of...such despair."

Analysis showed that at the start of the program, the students could be classified into two groups as a function of their "objective" descriptions. The first group was made up of students with an "objective" descriptive ability and included students with a concrete descriptive ability who struggled to speak about their inner world and integrate personal experiences. The second group had a greater "subjective" descriptive ability. It included students with an ability to express their inner world; however, their point of view was mainly projective, and their subjective experiences were at times perceived as objective. At the end of the program, the descriptive ability in both groups included both points of view. This suggests that work in the Open Studio and practicing phenomenological descriptive language while emphasizing the distinction between "objective" and "subjective" ultimately led to improved descriptive ability in both groups. This improvement made it possible to combine "objective" descriptions and "subjective" ones, thus creating a distinction between one student's point of view and that of another.

Self-efficacy. I also examined the contribution of work in the Open Studio on artworks to students' sense of self-efficacy. To measure this qualitatively, I used Bandura's (1986) theory and examined components he described as producing a self-efficacy experience: (a) personal achievements and failures from previous experiences; (b) indirect experience through observation of successes and failures of others' actions, and assessing the level of ability to complete a task or not in relation to others; (c) verbal persuasion, feedback and messages from meaningful figures in the context of self-efficacy and social influence; (d) physical and emotional awareness created in relation to an experience at times of success and failure.

From the interviews and reflective discourse, four categories were defined: (a) Students who described successful experiences and coping with various types of difficulties during work (work with materials, looking for and developing ideas, techniques, coping with expectations, desires, etc.). (b) Studio work in the presence of other students expanded efficacy. Students who were more self-confident demonstrated that it was possible to cope with problems, and other students tended to imitate them. For example, spreading plasticine on cardboard requires strength and consistency. Students watched the process and product and decided to work with it as well. (c) Discourse within the studio associated with verbal persuasion and meaningful figures, discourse that is neither critical nor judgmental, but phenomenological in describing qualities. The students talked about desires and thoughts which were validated by the art therapist. In this group, some students were leaders in the class. Receiving compliments or admiration from such students contributed to the experiences of self-efficacy and self-worth of other students. (d) Students' processing of emotional and physical reactions is predominantly the responsibility of the art therapists. They make sure that difficult emotional or physical experiences arising naturally in the studio are addressed and processed. One example of this is the disparity between what students saw in their imaginations and their actual artwork. This produced frustration, anger, jealousy and sometimes a desire to get rid of the artwork. The art therapist's reaction that focused on the experience enabled students to contain it, contributed to processing these experiences, and resolving the tension even when it was difficult to do so.

Summary and Conclusions

This chapter reviewed an Open Studio program adhering to a structured approach, "Bridge to Connection," implemented within a school framework. An Open Studio is based on the power of expression and healing in art and the creative processes. Individual work in the presence of a peer group allows students to locate themselves at the center of art exploration and have a platform to express the desires, ideas and works that represent them. The audience, which is made up of other students and art therapists, echoes the process from different points of view and add layers of artistic and social language to the process. Participation in the studio is voluntary. However, those who are interested in this framework are required to adhere to rules defining the therapeutic space and conduct.

The studio program is made up of a four-stage process, which provides a place for emotional experiences as part of the process of exploration, similar to an artist in an individual studio who expresses thoughts and emotions. Personal content is elicited throughout four consecutive stages: playful physical movement, projective work and creating metaphorical representations, artwork and verbal reflection. All these components help students structure their internal experience esthetically, clearly and in its entirety. The Open Studio program in its current form can also be applied for diverse therapeutic and educational purposes. Stages of the process can be channeled to any therapeutic goal such as working on regulation processes, improving conduct when coping with hurdles, etc.

Finally, a brief word to art therapists who decide work in an Open Studio where a different experience awaits them. You will find yourselves more creative and less an audience to others' creations. You will conduct eye-level discourse with your clients as artists to artists. You will learn to ask questions and mediate. You will postpone interpretation, be less worn out, play more and you will find yourselves happy for a day working in an Open Studio.

References

Bain, J.D., Ballantyne, R., Packer, J., & Mills, C. (1999). Using journal writing to enhance student teachers' reflectivity during field experience placements. *Teachers and Teaching: Theory and Practice*, *5*(1), 51–73.

Bandura, A. (1986). *Social foundations of thought and action: A social cognitive theory*. Englewood Cliffs, NJ: Prentice Hall.

Bandura, A. (1989). Regulation of cognitive processes through perceive self-efficacy. *Developmental Psychology*, *25*, 729–735.

Bandura, A. (1997). *Self-efficacy: The exercise of control*. New York: Freeman and Company.

Betensky, M. (1977). The phenomenological approach to art expression and art therapy. *Art Psychotherapy*, *4*, 173–179.

Betensky, M. (1995). *What do you see? Phenomenology of therapeutic art expression*. London: Jessica Kingsley Publishers.

Block, D., Harris, T., & Laing, S. (2005). Open studio process as a model of social action: a program for at-risk youth. *Art Therapy*, *22*(1), 32–38.

Boud, D.K., Keogh, R., & Walker, D. (2013). Promoting reflection in learning A modeli. *Boundaries of Adult Learning*, *1*, 32–57.

Boud, D.K., & Walker, R.D. (1985). *Reflection: turning experience into learning*. London: Kogan Page, 19.

Dewey, J. (1933). *How we think*. Boston, DC: Heath & Co.

Dewey, J. (1938). *Experience and education*. New York: Collier Macmillan.

Hazut, T.(2014). The "Haifa Approach" to art therapy. Methodology of perceptions and methods for organizing the therapeutic design and phenomenological investigation of processes and products. In R. Berger (Ed.), *Creation – the heart of therapy*. Kiryat Bialik: Ach Publications. (In Hebrew).

Heidegger, M. (1927). *Being and the time*. New York: Harper & Row

Heller, A. (2015). *The contribution of "Open Studio" program based experiential -learning to developing reflection abilities and self efficacy of elementary-school children*. (Doctoral dissertation). Babes Bolyai University, Romania.

Husserl, E. (1967). *Ideas*. London: Allen & Unwin.

Hyland Moon, C. (2002). *Studio art therapy*. London: Jessica Kingsley.

Kolb, D.A. (2014). Experiential learning as the science of learning and development. Englewood Cliffs, NJ: Prentice Hall.

Kramer, E. (2001). *Art as therapy: Collected papers*. Jessica Kingsley Publishers, London: Jessica Kingsley.

McNiff, S. (2000). *Art-based research*. London: Jessica Kingsley Publisher.

Moon, J.A. (2013). *Reflection in learning and professional development: Theory and practice*. London: Kogan Page.

Moustakas, C. (1994). *Phenomenological research methods*. Thousand Oaks, CA: Sage.

Schön, D.A. (1983). *The respective practitioner: How professionals think in action*. New York: Basic Books.

Zohar, T. (2004). Student-teachers in reflection processes: An integrative and interactive model. In S. Guri-Rosenblit (Ed.), *Teachers in a world of change: Trends and challenges* (pp. 298–321). Ra'anana: Open University of Israel. (In Hebrew).

8 A Dialectic Model for Art Therapy with Students Who Behave Aggressively

Edna Nissimov-Nahum

Introduction

Maor's confrontational appearance was deceiving. At first glance he seemed strong, assertive and determined, but he was in fact hiding his pain, which often left adults feeling helpless, frustrated and angry. His behavior, which was locked in a destructive loop, challenged the educational system to find effective solutions. When the extensive educational response to Maor's behavior did not bring about change, he was referred for individual art therapy. Maor's parents and the school staff had clear expectations to put an end to his aggression and provide him and his parents with relief so that Maor could develop like his peers. Before accepting him for therapy, I considered the many issues involved. How would I create a secure relationship with him when he displayed defiant, confrontational and distancing behavior? How would art help him to express himself even though he feared it? How would I get assistance from his parents and teachers when they themselves felt helpless? How would I, in my role as an art therapist, contain him when he elicited my personal experiences of aggression and victimization? These expectations and challenges made me flinch, but I was curious and felt highly motivated to treat Maor.

This chapter is based on a dialectic model deriving from studies that have examined the practice, dilemmas, achievements and difficulties that art therapists deal with in educational settings (Nissimov-Nahum, 2007; 2013). It discusses a range of approaches to aggression as a function of the variety of external and internal factors that drive it and the many challenges that characterize the treatment of this type of behavior. The model is intended to help address and deal with the specific challenges that arise when encountering and treating individuals who display aggressiveness (Nissimov-Nahum, 2008). It is illustrated by a case study that shows how the model is implemented.

Theoretical Background

The Dialectic Model for Art Therapy with Aggressive Students provides an adaptable response to extreme behaviors and presents clear principles for the integration of art therapy with psychodynamic, emotional, cognitive, behavioral, systemic and familial components. The model presented in Figure 8.1 highlights two aspects of the role of art therapists: the spaces for intervention (ellipses) and the focal points for intervention (arrows).

The dialectic model presents three intervention spaces (Nissimov-Nahum, 2008). The *interpersonal space*, which relates to the relationship between the art therapist and the client, is the central workspace that exists on a weekly basis. However, in order to improve the quality of therapy, it is crucial to simultaneously open the gateways to two other spaces. As part of the *systemic space*, the art therapist is required to make a meaningful connection with other individuals in the student's life, such as teachers and parents, to increase the impact of the therapeutic process on the student's life. In addition, when working with this population, the therapist needs to deal with his/her personal experiences of aggression courageously and therefore is forced to take a deeper look into the *personal space* as well. According to this model, simultaneously working in the three spaces is essential for the effectiveness of the therapeutic process. However, there is risk involved, since within each of the spaces separately, and often in all of them together, an immense level of tension can arise due to the challenges faced by the art therapist during the multidimensional encounter with aggression.

In terms of the focal points of intervention, the principle that should guide the art therapist in the three different spaces is *acceptance* and the *direction for change*. Working according to this principle will help overcome the tension in the three spaces by creating a space of acceptance in response to the emotional experience that the client needs, the individuals in the client's environment and even the therapist him or herself need, but also in directing them to achieve change. This principle may be perceived as an internal contradiction where acceptance may appear to be the opposite of

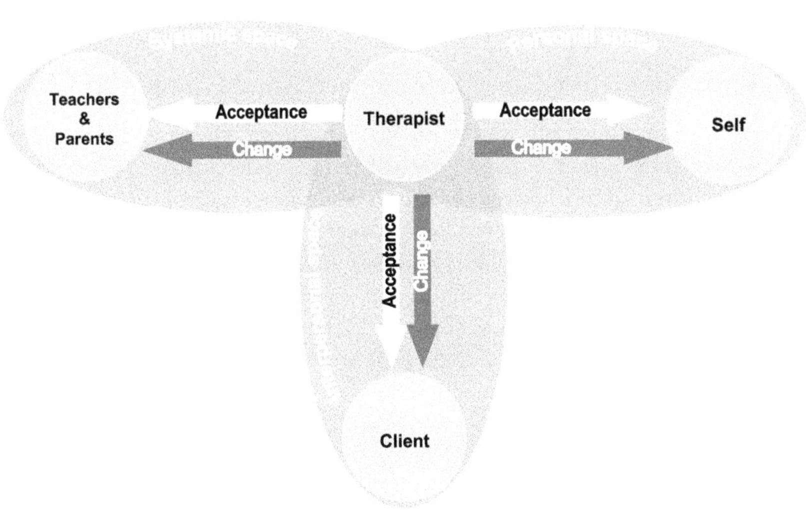

Figure 8.1 The Dialectic Model: the Roles of the Art Therapist Working with Students Who Behave Aggressively.

the intended change. How can you accept someone and try to change him/her simultaneously? However, it should be noted that the components of the principle, which seem to be contradictory, are dialectically linked to one another in that each strengthens and completes the other. As such, a relationship of acceptance can foster change. When the client feels accepted, understood and appreciated, he/she may agree to give up destructive elements and begin to believe in change. On the other hand, when directed towards change, the client realizes that acceptance does not indicate compliance with aggressive behavior, but instead offers a more effective way of solving problems in an empathic manner. The novel experience of significant acceptance by the art therapist of the student, the student's teachers and his/her parents, as well as the student's own experiences can present an opportunity for more flexible solutions. Nevertheless, conveying a sense of acceptance is not sufficient to convert aggressive behavior into adaptive behavior. It is therefore important to concurrently adopt an approach that encourages change.

This chapter presents the application of this model through the description of a clinical example about an individual art therapy process. It is discussed in terms of the spaces of the model, and the intervention focal points are highlighted within each space. It also outlines the assessment process at the start of the therapeutic process (which includes observations, obtaining background information, conversations with the teachers and meetings with the parents), as well as the specific tools that are most appropriate to this model (figure drawing, the six-part story method, family drawings, defining central issues, anger drawings and an event-processing conversation). This is followed by depictions of interventions from the therapeutic process that illustrate their integration into the dialectic model.

Description of the Working Model and a Clinical Example

Maor was about ten years old when we started art therapy. During my observation in his classroom and after receiving some background information, which mainly touched on his aggression and resistance, I noticed that he was agitated, easily distracted, and struggled to control himself, accept rules and follow instructions. His external appearance conveyed rage. His behavior revealed difficulties listening, prolonging gratification and staying motivated not to give up. However, he touched my heart. His eyes revealed him to be a sensitive, intelligent and creative student, but also an introverted and closed individual.

The Personal Space (The Therapist's Experiences)

Treating students who behave aggressively often elicits complex feelings in art therapists who work to contain, accept and help clients, but may feel threatened by the intensity of their aggressive behavior. Therapists often feel fear, anger, rejection and even identification with the situation and may respond by distancing themselves from the client, fighting back, feeling helpless and also submission. The level of tension may also be aggravated during their encounters with teachers and parents. Therapists may feel angry, blame and criticize them as a result of their over-identification with the student's anger. Alternatively, therapists may identify with the teachers' and/or parents' positions and blame the student for not changing. The tumultuous experiences that these clients elicit, particularly when confronted with unprocessed issues from the therapists' personal world, may cause a loss of appropriate professional distancing and therapeutic responses that do not meet the clients' needs.

Maor evoked intense feelings within me and for this reason I chose to use the language of art when I entered my therapy room to review the observation process. I wanted to better understand the visible and hidden aspects of my perceptions of the relationship. I used the drawing task technique described in Nissimov-Nahum (2009), which suggests drawing two images on one page that metaphorically represent the client and the therapist and their relationship. This serves to discover, beyond words and the conscious level, the hidden aspects of the therapeutic relationship. It was created for use in research, supervision and therapy to assess the contribution of art to a better understanding of the personal space according to the dialectic model (Nissimov-Nahum, 2009). In this case, as an art therapist, it enabled me to more accurately *accept* and understand my perceptions of the relationship that was about to be formed, and the questions that arose as a result led to a *change* in my internal perceptions of the therapeutic process, as described below.

Maor was depicted as a curled-up turtle-snail, and I was drawn as a wholesome loaf of bread. The images were equal in size, close to each other and similar in color, but I noticed that they belonged to different worlds: the dynamic animal world versus the static world of food. Undoubtedly, the turtle-snail hints at the protective armor and the slow progress that is required in this therapeutic process, and the loaf of bread may be a response to the emotional hunger that I felt emanating from him. However, as I looked at the drawing, several questions arose. First, when depicting Maor as a turtle-snail, what represented his aggression? Was I identifying with his introverted side and denying his aggression? Second, concerning our relationship, whereas a turtle-snail eats plants and vegetables, why did I offer him a loaf of bread? Did he need different and more suitable food? Third, with respect to my role as a therapist: Why did I offer him inappropriate food? Was our relationship destined to be barren and frustrating because he would not need me if I were a loaf of bread? Why did I choose such a passive image? Was the sense of incompatibility projected onto me from his world? Or did it originate from my world and was transferred to him?

The Systemic Space (Therapist-Teacher-Parent Relationship)

Art therapy within the educational system is conducted differently than in other settings because it operates in the environment in which the aggressive behavior is most prevalent. The school staff, together with the parents, are involved in the process of referral to art therapy which typically occurs following considerable effort but failure to address the problem by the school. Art therapists, who typically meet with their clients once a week, can increase their influence by working with teachers and parents who have daily interactions with the students. The adults who are present in the students' lives have numerous opportunities to immediately and directly respond to the student's aggressive behavior. In many cases, they may handle it appropriately, but in some cases, they unintentionally maintain the aggressive behavior. Conversely, when the therapists remove the teacher and the parents from the therapeutic setting, they may develop an over-identification with the client and criticize the adults present in the student's life, thus reducing the likelihood of making a positive contribution to the therapeutic process. Furthermore, the therapists may create a split in the student's life by making it difficult to implement the changes in perceptions and behaviors that were experienced in the therapy room in other settings. When teachers and parents are not included in the therapeutic process, they may convey conflicting messages about it and inadvertently impair the student's response to therapy.

The dialectic model aims to create a systemic alliance. I suggest that after obtaining background information, observing and speaking with the teacher, the beginning of the therapeutic process should include three sessions with the parents, as described below. Experience teaches us that despite the difficulties involved in meeting with parents while their child is being treated in an educational setting, the effort is beneficial and not only helps to build a solid foundation for therapy, but also contributes to changes in the child's environment (Nissimov-Nahum, 2008).

First session. During the first session with Maor's parents, which was intended to get acquainted with them and obtain more information, they were disturbed by Maor's frequent refusals to go to school and expressed concern about his studies given the extreme tension between him and the educational staff. When I asked what was behind this tension, they described Maor's aggression as taking over his entire existence. He resorted to physical violence against property, students and adults (teachers and the school principal) indiscriminately. They mentioned that he had been diagnosed as a child as having a learning disability and an Attention Deficit Hyperactivity Disorder.

I saw that the parents loved Maor and cared for him, but that they also felt helpless. They also seemed out of touch with reality. Although they claimed that there were not many difficulties at home, it is evident that they were struggling with parental authority and had problems in their relationship. His mother typically gave in to his demands, but his father reacted aggressively and punished him. Their distress and unsettled feelings, which ranged from shame to genuine concern, apparently prompted them to seek help from the school staff.

During our conversation, Maor's parents painfully told me that their son sometimes cried and revealed that he was afraid of himself. I assumed that Maor's fear of his own anger and aggression was related to his feeling that he and his parents were losing control over the situation. I inquired about expressions of anger in the family and learned that his paternal grandfather was violent and Maor's tantrums reminded Maor's father of his own father. This often made Maor's father feel helpless, and explained why he reacted so strongly to such behavior. His mother said that Maor resembled her in his impulsive responses, and that she got impatient with him and responded in an unsuitable manner to his behavior. She was pessimistic about his ability to change as a result of her experiences with her brother who has a psychiatric disorder, and therefore said that she gives in to Maor's demands. It is therefore understandable why they refused to treat him medically. The parents' personal experiences, which they shared with candor during the first session, explained their despair and lack of motivation regarding their son. I realized that a vicious circle was developing in their family in which the more Maor sensed his parents' despair, the more closed within himself he became and expressed more anger, which occasionally erupted and which heightened his parents' despair. During the session, I was aware of my inner struggle that alternated between waves of criticism and anger towards Maor's parents' behavior and feelings of empathy and sympathy for the challenges that they were facing. I mentioned that given Maor's difficulties, I understood their love for him and greatly appreciated their determination to pursue help. In addition, I described my work plan and emphasized that in order to help Maor, it was important that the adults present in his life should make a meaningful connection and work together to alleviate his difficulties. These two statements illustrate the beginning of the application of the dialectic principle in the relationship with Maor's parents: I demonstrated *acceptance* through empathy, yet I also pushed towards a process of *change.*

Second session. The second session took place after an initial conversation with Maor's teacher that we both initiated. We started by conveying a clear message to the parents that was both supportive and *accepting* which would help them be empathetic to Maor's difficulties and reduce their feelings of guilt as well as Maor's. We presented an explanation for Maor's aggression in which we referred to his frustration as a result of the considerable gap between his potential and his weak performance, which stemmed from his diagnosed learning disabilities, Attention Deficit Hyperactivity Disorder and his difficulty articulating his feelings and seeking help from adults out of his lack of trust. His immense frustration and low self-esteem were reflected in his anger and aggression, which was also projected at his peers and limited his social interactions. We also explained that Maor's problems could be addressed and changed based on our experiences with similar students, thus conveying to his parents that they were not alone in their predicament or in dealing with Maor's aggression. In addition, we recommended that for a trial period, they would reconsider administering his medications, which contributed to his impaired self-esteem, suffering and poor academic performance. In this way, we offered them hope for *change*. We also asked them to accept our shared responsibility from the start of the therapeutic process. This appeared to provide some degree of tranquility, instilled hope and reduced their feelings of isolation and helplessness.

Third session. The third session reinforced the supportive conditions and was the first session where Maor was present. His parents explained to him that they had decided to try a therapeutic intervention and in so doing expressed profound recognition of the connection that we had formed. I appreciated their decision and invited them to make a joint drawing in the art therapy room. The purpose of the session was to deliver the message that we could enjoy ourselves together and that we acknowledged the family's behavioral patterns.

Maor entered shyly and hid behind his mother. His sense of tension and rage could be felt without any words being spoken. When I offered him a plastic cup of water, he crushed it until it lost its shape. He rejected my invitation to take part in the joint drawing task, turned his back on me and walked towards the shelf of toys. I recognized Maor's lack of hope and confidence, as well as his difficulty adapting to new situations. I agreed with his choice (*acceptance*) and when he took a box of animals to the table, I was impressed with his initiative and suggested that everyone choose an animal for themselves. Maor chose a big black shark, his father chose a black horse and his mother chose a small, smiling, friendly dolphin. Maor was the only one who noticed that the horse had no ears, smiled shyly and whispered that the horse could not hear. When I suggested they create a surrounding environment for the animals, they drew pouring rain and a stormy sea. In the story that I suggested we put in writing, the father wanted to tame the sharks, but Maor declined. He sunk the boat and his shark devoured the people. His mother attempted to rescue them with the dolphin, but Maor said no, and added a flying dragon to help the shark eat everyone. Maor wanted to bury them at sea, but when he saw his parents' astonished expressions, he agreed to save them.

Art making not only enabled *acceptance* and enjoyment during the joint drawing task, but also strengthened the understanding of the family narrative and enhanced the family relationships and communication patterns through the hands-on activity. The joint drawing helped Maor and his parents get acquainted with me and with the creative and therapeutic language. His parents discovered Maor's creative abilities and strengthened their commitment to their role in therapy. I gained a better understanding of the family dynamics that were both visible and hidden. The power of the joint drawing left a mark on me: I felt Maor's anger at the world as well as his parents' desperate attempts to regulate it. However, Maor managed to communicate his aggression carefully and was contained and protected when he expressed his anger. Maor's sense of his father's lack of attentiveness and the lack of boundary setting reflected his needs to his father. At the same time, his mother appeared to be close to Maor (they both chose sea animals), but the small size and vulnerability of the dolphin reflected her weakness and the complexity of their relationship.

According to the model and after the joint drawing task, I told Maor that his parents had met with me and told me about him and his family. I admired his skills as they were described by his parents (*acceptance*), but I spoke about him and his parents' difficulty coping with anger (*direction for change*). I explained that his aggression was a way of telling us how difficult it was for him. I suggested that the two of us meet every week and establish a relationship that would involve playing and working with art materials, but we would also address expressions of anger and aggression. In this way, I communicated the goals of art therapy to the family; namely, to reduce the level of aggression and improve Maor's interpersonal relationships with friends, parents and teachers. From their reactions, I saw that they were relieved and reassured. Despite their difficulties directly discussing the issues, I assumed that they were in the "Contemplation" stage (Prochaska, Norcross, & DiClemente, 1994) where they were aware of the problem even if they were not yet ready for change. There seemed to be a two-pronged attitude in that they showed interest, but had not identified the path to change. In this case, the teacher had already reached the "Preparation" stage, where she took responsibility, and was ready to adapt to Maor to generate the process of change.

The Interpersonal Space (Client-Therapist Relationship)

The special relationship that develops during therapy has a crucial impact on its quality and outcomes. Establishing trust is critical in every therapeutic process, but is essential with clients who are referred for therapy for aggressive behavior without consulting them first. This behavior, which reflects rejection, anger, frustration and disappointment with interpersonal relationships, can make it difficult to connect despite the secure and protected environment of the art therapy room. Furthermore, the artwork during art therapy, which may serve as a sublimative space for expressing aggression and as a safe container for anger, can backfire because of the aggression and threaten the therapist and the entire room. In certain situations, this may create a rift between the frustrated aggression in the reality of the client's life and the situation in the therapy room, which may be unable to allow for overt aggression or verbalizations of it.

The dialectic model outlines a way to address these challenges. *Acceptance* is realized through the warm relationship and the creative abundance as a platform for expression, understanding the client and the establishment of closeness. *Change* is manifested by sharing the goals of therapy with the client, outlining the therapeutic contract and limiting expressions of aggression, interventions during the creative work in relation to the end product and by encouraging empathy towards others. The interventions related to aggression inside and outside the therapy room involve authoritative responses, learning physical relaxation techniques and conversations to process the event (Nissimov-Nahum, 2008).

Messages of warmth, support and genuine interest in Maor's needs were crucial in establishing the therapeutic relationship, particularly due to his closed nature, internalized rage and despondency about receiving help. As expected, the relationship with Maor began with the testing of boundaries. He spoke very little but agreed to play and create. During the first session, I spoke to him about our contract using the dialectic principle: *Acceptance* was made possible through my willingness to make a permanent, continuous and containing relationship that allowed for expression and pleasure, and the *direction for change* was expressed through limiting his aggression with regards to the therapeutic relationship and materials in the therapy room. Each session started by asking him to describe a pleasant and an unpleasant experience that had happened during the week in order to help him express himself and create connections between reality and art therapy. The trust and security in our relationship was established gradually and primarily using art-based interventions that allowed him to express his inner world more and more.

Despite the intimidating depiction, in our therapeutic bubble Maor turned out to be a pleasant and sensitive student. He came to art therapy willingly and consistently and skipped joyfully on his way from the classroom. In the room he exhibited introverted behavior, replied briefly to simple questions and took time to think before answering. He often shrugged his shoulders to signal that either he did not know how to answer or was not interested, and it seemed it was difficult to express his needs in words. I therefore gave him several choices of activities in our sessions and validated his choices and wishes.

When Maor asked me to suggest the subject of his drawings, he revealed his fear of free expression, his difficulty with failure and his low self-esteem. He may have even feared a situation in which unconscious content would be expressed uncontrollably. I suggested he make guided drawings to help him tell his story. These included how he perceived himself (the six-part story making) and the relationships within his family (family drawing).

The six-part story making (Lahad, 2000a). I suggested that Maor create a story-drawing on a sheet of paper that is folded into six parts. I used the projective technique that combines a verbal aspect with the artwork to illustrate his inner perceptions of these beliefs, feelings, thoughts, conflicts, coping abilities and modes of communication in an indirect, safe way. After each of my questions and in the order of the folded page, Maor drew inside one of the folds and upon completion he was given the next question. The questions were: Who is the main character? What is the role or task of the character? Who or what can help the character fulfill the mission? Who or what can hinder the character from fulfilling the mission? How will the character deal with this? What happens at the end? Maor complied and enjoyed the task. After creating the drawing in stages, he stated:

> The main character is Spiderman. His mission is to help people. He saves people from the bad guys, hangs from his web and that's how he doesn't get hurt. The bad guys constantly bother him. Spiderman always has important missions and he doesn't even sleep. The monkey helps him a lot and Spiderman saved him because he can't climb fast. Spiderman is very strong, he doesn't cry, and overcomes everything and all problems. Spiderman helps everyone and saves them.

Maor chose a familiar superhero story, probably to make it easier for himself. Through identification with the protagonist, he presented a position of stability, took responsibility for saving others and sacrificed himself for them. Like the superhero, he does not reveal his weakness and is forced to face complex challenges. However, Maor's drawing of Spiderman was only a skeleton because it was transparent, empty, had no hands, a fake smile, and showed weakness and helplessness. The hero, who is supposed to rescue and help people, is portrayed in the drawing as handicapped and incapable of performing his many rescue missions. The main character is alone on every mission, and even his assistant needs to be rescued because he cannot climb. Thus, the immense gap between the wish for "a very strong Spiderman" and his appearance as handicapped and missing two arms appeared to reveal Maor's ambivalence and insecurities about his own skills. This was also expressed in his intense need to be admired and validated verbally and in writing during the therapeutic sessions. I painfully observed the gap between the story that was told and the character that was drawn. It revealed the difference between what he wanted and what was obtainable: Maor's fragile inner perception, characterized by weakness and vulnerability, was hiding behind his strong (forceful) and false (the empty smile) appearance.

Family drawing. When I asked Maor to draw his family, he hesitated because he did not know how to draw their bodies, but he accepted the challenge when I suggested he could draw images that reflected them. He began by drawing images of many of his family members (uncles, cousins, grandparents), as though he was justifying their importance in his life, but also as a way to reject his difficulty in dealing with his nuclear family. He then drew his little sister as a princess, his mother beside her as a cellphone and his father on the other side as the letter X with scales. He then declared that he was finished. After admiring the many interesting images that he created, I mentioned that he had not drawn himself. He was surprised to learn this and thought for a long time about what image to create for himself. I understood this as his difficulty to find a clear identity and a safe place within his family. In the end he drew a small flame in the corner of the page far away from his nuclear family. When talking about the images, we pointed out their differences in size, their proximity and the content. We noted the special features of each one: a sister who is raised like a princess, but looks more like a threatening ghost figure, a mother who speaks to the entire world, but struggles to listen to Maor, a father who thinks he knows everything, but constantly criticizes Maor, and finally Maor's fire that seems weak, but is burning and threatening from the sidelines to burn up the other images in a blaze. The map of the family relationship that Maor created revealed his experiences within the family and indicated that his parents put his sister on a pedestal, whereas he was pushed to the sidelines with his anger and loneliness.

I thought that Maor had a secret he had locked away about himself. He felt lonely and misunderstood, was failing in school and unsuccessful in his life. He was apparently not only disappointing himself but also his parents, friends and teachers. In his solitude, he tried as hard as he could to lock his secret away. Occasionally, the distress erupted uncontrollably and with such great anger that he frightened himself, just like the other students who were afraid of him and distanced themselves from him. Adults became furious with him and lost hope.

The central issue. At the end of the assessment stage, I contemplated the central issue related to Maor's deep emotional pain. I hypothesized that his main conflict was related to poor as compared to realistic self-esteem and that the key emotions were sadness and anger. In Mann's approach, the therapist should formulate the client's central issue while considering four elements: support (the clients' strengths and abilities), time (when the problem started and erupted), self-attitude (the clients' perception of the self in relation to the pain) and emotion (the central emotion that the client reflects), to which I usually add a fifth component – the symptomatic behavior observed in reality (Mann, 1973; Nissimov-Nahum, 2013). The formulation of the central issue helped me better understand the processes that led Maor to feel distress and strike out at his surroundings:

> You are a clever and sensitive child, with the ability and will to succeed and progress (support). However, in recent years (time) you feel that you are not being listened to, and the efforts you make to deal with your difficulties are not appreciated (self-attitude). Therefore, you feel "undeserving," worthless, sad and angry (emotion). Your difficulty in articulating these experiences causes you to act aggressively at times (behavior).

Initially I was able to talk to Maor about the central issue indirectly using the images from the drawings, but gradually it was also introduced directly.

I also continued to think about him in terms of the central issue. It helped me help him to understand himself and allow him to feel more understood. In my conversations with his teacher and parents, I used the definition of the central issue to interpret his inner world. The simple phrasing helped them understand his pain and aggressive behavior.

Creating freely. As the relationship developed, Maor felt brave enough to choose the subjects for his drawings. They mostly reflected anger, such as a child lighting a large bonfire which could potentially burn a house down, or a drawing of a giant, evil warrior who threatens little planet Earth. At a later stage, his drawings reflected feelings of loneliness, such as an empty palace where no one wants to live, or a solitary tree that was in danger because it was neglected.

Drawing the anger. Maor started a ritual that he carried out at the beginning of each session: he swung on the swing in the art therapy room and punched the punching bag. These actions alleviated his tensions regarding our relationship and enabled a space to discuss important issues. While on the swing during one of the sessions, Maor told me that he had not gone to school the previous week because he was afraid of his outbursts of anger in the classroom. This indicated that Maor felt comfortable talking about his concerns, but that he was also motivated to get help and improve his self-control. I asked what his anger looked like. He described it as "a tsunami that reaches all the way to the galaxies." When he agreed to draw his anger, I mentioned that to me his anger looked "huge, powerful, inundating and threatening to destroy anything in its path." When we spoke about the drawing, I commented: "Sometimes it seems that the tsunami will never end, but anger, just like any wave, peaks and then descends, breaks and subsides." By addressing the undulating pattern of anger, I was implying a motif of change.

Often, we swung the punching bag at each other forcefully and developed an angry discussion in gibberish. This way Maor had a space to express his anger at a very high intensity, but also shielded himself from visible and direct content. We built up a story about a king and prince who were angry with each other because the king refused to give the prince a cellphone. This story largely reflected one of the most frequent conflicts between him and his father. The phone could signify a status symbol, but also Maor's longing for a connection.

During one of the sessions, Maor threw the punching bag at me hard. I understood that an aggressive fight was developing, and I could relate to the threat felt by his friends, parents and teachers. When I was under threat of becoming a victim, which I considered intolerable, I reminded him of our contract and our boundaries in therapy which permit the expression of anger through movement and play, but without harming anyone. I asked Maor directly if he was angry with me and he struggled to confess. I told him that his aggression towards me with the punching bag indicated that he was angry. I encouraged him to share the anger with me and remarked that the anger symbolized a red traffic light that protects him from danger, so it was important to pay attention to it. He reconciled and said that he was angry at me for missing the previous art therapy session. We saw how his aggression concealed the anger which further hid his disappointment. I acknowledged his disappointment and expressed regret that he had not been informed, and had waited for a long time before returning to his classroom.

Conversation to process an event. After several sessions when I inquired about his absence from art therapy the week before, he answered shyly that he had been suspended for two days from school. At that stage in therapy, we had developed a good relationship, but expressions of anger and aggression were mostly conveyed non-verbally. I felt that this event created an opportunity to expand the treatment of aggressive outbursts to verbal means and I chose to use the "Event-Processing Conversation" method (Nissimov-Nahum, 2008). This method consists of five stages and was designed to help Maor perceive the sequence and context of his behavior, as well as process his inner experiences in these situations (*acceptance*) while observing the attitudes of others and finding more suitable solutions (*change*). When I asked him: "What happened?" (Stage 1), Maor looked down and remained silent. I reflected that I understood it was difficult for him to tell me and suggested that he choose art materials to create with.

He took a lump of clay, flattened it and kneaded it continually without giving it a definable shape. He used a pair of scissors to stab the lump hard from every angle. When the entire lump was pierced, he asked if he could keep the "anger" moist, protected and locked in a closed container. When I inquired about the appearance of his anger, he answered: "My anger is like my heart, burning with flames and avoiding eruption." Maor did not allow the lump to dry as though he wanted to maintain the possibility of allowing the anger to "live on" and control or change it; i.e., reduce, enlarge, cover or paint it. Only after touching the material did Maor begin to tell the story:

> We were playing ball during recess and the kids threw the ball at me. I caught it but I dropped it. One of the kids cursed me because I didn't catch the ball. It was noisy and chaotic, and I couldn't hear what they were saying to me. The kids decided to take me out of the game. I ran after the boy and hit him. Another boy went to report me to the teacher in charge. She didn't listen to me, she just grabbed me, so I kicked her to let me go and ran away.

First, I showed empathy and told Maor that I understood that he had kicked the teacher out of his distress. He felt that she was not listening to him, he felt lonely and humiliated, so he attacked her. Maor opened his eyes in amazement when he realized that I was not reprimanding him for his behavior. The experience of *acceptance* and acknowledging his feelings helped me to continue the process and guide us towards *change*.

When I asked him: "What boundaries were crossed?" (Stage 2), he replied: "I know I shouldn't hit students and teachers. Believe me I didn't mean to do it, it just came out of me." I responded to him: "I believe every word you said. Now that you're calm, it might be worthwhile to find out: What did you feel in your body? How did you feel? What were you thinking about? (Stage 3). Maor felt the pain physically throughout his body like sharp, painful stabs. He ran his hand up and down his body to demonstrate how the pain wriggled over his body. He thought that he was being attacked, that no one sees, listens or understands him. I thought to myself that at that moment, Maor felt insignificant, vulnerable and anxious, and tried to defend himself against these feelings through aggression. He claimed that this pattern repeats itself: no one listens to him, but they listen to the other side. Together we attempted to understand the pain that he feels when others do not take him into account. His feeling of rejection was so strong when the children tried to take him out of the game because he felt insignificant, unworthy and afraid of being isolated. Our conversation touched on Maor's chronic pain and was accompanied by tears. I reminded him of the family drawing and we noticed that this experience repeated itself at home and also elicited aggression there.

After Maor sensed that I understood and accepted him, I continued to navigate towards change by clarifying other people's perspectives. I asked Maor: "How does the boy who is being attacked feel? How does the teacher feel?" (Stage 4). Maor found it difficult to empathize with their pain and became barricaded inside his own world. I decided to share and consider the positions of the boy who was disappointed that the ball dropped during the game, the boy who asked for help from the teacher in charge because he was worried and the position of the teacher who wanted to calm him down and solve the problem. I commented that it is often difficult for us to perceive the situation from the viewpoint of another individual, and although he feels attacked, it is not sure that in this case someone really wanted to intentionally attack him. The series of events led to the complex situation. It is possible that even for a single event, all the parties involved perceived it differently. Empathy, even if it develops through a cognitive process, is essential to understanding the perspective of others, and in developing a sense of support from others that is absent in aggressive behavior. Finally, I asked Maor: "What can be done to resolve the situation?" (Stage 5). This is an important stage, which is intended for practical implementation in the therapeutic process. We talked about how he could recognize anger in his body before it erupts, how he could calm himself, move away, seek help when he feels anger, unfair treatment or being overlooked. We also concluded that in our conversations with his parents and teacher, we could communicate the association between his lack of attention and his anger, which is expressed frantically through aggressive outbursts. In this way, we established a connection between art therapy and reality, and between Maor's inner world and those of the adults who are responsible for him.

Combining Spaces: the Systemic and the Interpersonal

The relationships that I developed with the school staff during Maor's therapeutic process were significant. I gave two lectures and workshops during the academic year. In the first one, an explanation and demonstration of art therapy, I emphasized the importance of a professional relationship between arts therapists and the educational staff when the therapy takes place in the education system. In the second lecture, I addressed different approaches to dealing with anger that I taught through my own experience, using the structure of the "Event-Processing Conversation" method. The joint meetings between all parties involved in Maor's therapy were needed to strengthen the *acceptance* in the relationship and to steer towards the required *change*.

Joint session: The teacher and Maor. One of the benefits of treating clients within the education system is the opportunity to expand the impact of art therapy through continuous, frequent and casual discussions with the teacher. During these conversations, I listened to Maor's teacher and adopted the dialectic principle with respect to our relationship, but also when relating to Maor. I was impressed by her sensitivity and willingness to understand and help him, and I even suggested ways of coping with the challenges. After "translating" Maor's internal world for her through an explanation of the central issue, she was moved by the content that emerged and implemented the objective. She strengthened her relationship with Maor, listened to him, respected and valued his efforts (*acceptance*), but at the same time was authoritative when needed, limited the level of aggression in class and helped him perceive others better. She also encouraged him to control himself and to find more flexible solutions to dealing with everyday challenges (*change*) (Nissimov-Nahum, 2008).

Subsequently, I accepted Maor's request to invite her to the art therapy room. She was impressed by his drawings and this filled him with excitement. They set a regular time during the week to meet together and to share a good and a bad experience, where if necessary, she would offer help. Maor apparently felt *acceptance* because of her readiness to listen to him, and he felt secure enough within the relationship to share his difficulties with her to *change* his attitude.

Joint session: The parents and Maor. Both parents came to school during the middle of a workday for the fourth session despite the problem of finding time in their busy schedules. This demonstrated an appreciation of the significance of art therapy and their continued commitment to Maor. I also presented the central issue to them to help them understand their son. They were able to understand the connection between life events and Maor's feelings, thoughts and behavior. However, they did not know how to overcome these difficulties and I noted that they were not yet available to genuinely listen to him. I suggested that they devote more thought to his experiences (mentalization) and establish routine channels of communication close to dinner time or before bed. I also asked them to attend another joint session with Maor.

During the joint session – the fifth session with the parents – they complained that Maor was spending a great deal of time playing computer games at home. I learned that Maor's parents had shift work that required them to be absent from home for long periods. I stated that I understood Maor's behavior, who was trying to fill his time alone with an interesting activity (*acceptance* of Maor), but I also agreed with his parents that extended periods of time in front of the computer were not good for him (*acceptance* of the parents). In doing so, we defined a space of listening and mutual acceptance. Together we explored strategies for *change*. The mother decided to talk to him over the phone when he came home from school and send him encouraging text messages, and in return he would make sure to stop playing on the computer when one of the parents came home to engage and interact together. The parents promised to put their telephones aside, at least during dinner, when the family members would talk about their day's experiences.

Maor also had the courage to complain: "Mom and Dad are always busy, even on Saturdays, and I go out alone to ride my bike." His mother did not understand the context, but here I learned that since they moved to a different apartment, Maor had been separated from many people he knew, and he particularly missed one family in his old neighborhood with whom he was very close. The joint session enabled the family members to become closer because they engaged with each other by listening and *accepting*, and also gave Maor space to talk about his strong internal content. The parents assured me that a *change* would occur that would allow them to spend time with their children and relieve Maor's feelings of abandonment.

The Personal Space

My drawing from the beginning of the therapeutic process preoccupied me for a long time. I was particularly bothered by the fact that the turtle-snail image had overlooked Maor's aggressive behavior and identified with his introverted side. I also thought about the passive perspective of my role in the image of the loaf of bread. I realized that I have gotten into a trap of over-acceptance and avoidance of intended change (Nissimov-Nahum, 2009). Due to my identification with his experience of rejection and sense of victimization, there was a risk that I could have denied his difficulties expressed through his aggression and its implications. In this case, Maor, his parents and his teachers would not get a suitable therapeutic response.

As I observed Maor's drawing in the "Six-part Story Method," I understood why I had identified. The transparency of the figures in the drawing also conveyed my personal experience of being "invisible." During my childhood and until my late adolescence, I felt that I served as an emotional container for the expectations, wishes, adjustments and demands of the people around me. However, no one, including myself, inquired, referred to or showed interest in what "I wanted." As a girl who wanted to please others, I understood that this was the way to feel a sense of belonging and be loved. I was determined to excel and succeed for my parents' sake. I often overlooked my own needs in order to please others and earn their approval and love. Fortunately, since then, I have learned exactly what "I want" and have followed my own inclinations, but I confess that I often get caught up in the debate: "Should I give up or do what I want even at the expense of those around me?"

This insight, which alerted me to the risks involved in therapy, motivated me to search for other images. The image that I redrew to represent Maor was a turtle-snail with porcupine quills. It was evident that the quills were protecting the turtle-snail from harm. While I was searching for an image for myself, I thought about what Maor needed from me, and about my active approach in therapy. I wanted to choose an animal that could create a sense of closeness between these worlds, and therefore chose the image of a guide dog. This animal is characterized by strength and composure, and conveys a message of warmth, attentiveness and assistance, but is firm enough not to be intimidated by the porcupine's quills. The ability to play with the images and adapt them helped me understand the difficulties that could sabotage the therapeutic process and overcome them by understanding the aggression and the emotional content that it masked and being present to help overcome Maor's difficulties.

Summary and Conclusions

When referred to art therapy for his aggression and difficulties expressing himself, Maor not only created a smokescreen that concealed his deep-seated vulnerabilities, but also provided clues that dissipated the smoke and provided hints as to ways to help others understand his aggression. In fact, how can one be aware and acknowledge that the parents, despite their love for him, in fact ignored him, felt disappointed and were unavailable? Even in children's stories, the wolf is permitted to devour the grandmother, but the rejecting mother is typically a stepmother. Maor developed an aggression mechanism to deal with his pain. The artwork provided a pathway into his unconscious world, but the verbal expression – through metaphorical stories and direct conversations – made it possible to understand and reveal the content. As the relationship developed, the connection between the artwork and verbal communication became stronger and the connection between his inner and outer worlds intensified. In my opinion, the artwork and the verbal communication could not have existed separately. Their combination paved the way towards an understanding of the meaning.

The active approach that I chose to use was an example of the application of the dialectic approach. In the *interpersonal space* the focused dynamic approach presented the foundation for understanding the sources of the problem, defining the central issue and establishing the relationship between us. This relationship withstood many challenges and enabled Maor to feel understood, protected and significant. Maor's turbulent feelings were alleviated. The direction for change was accomplished through the processing of anger and changing his attitudes towards himself and those around him. The discussions on situations outside the art therapy room helped improve Maor's coping abilities and form a connection between therapy and reality. From his low initial point of hating school, Maor's self-esteem improved, he began to believe in himself and his capabilities, managed to express himself and deal with difficulties in a flexible manner. From a state in which his classmates were afraid of him and distanced themselves from him, Maor was able to make more meaningful connections and thrive socially.

This process was also supported by the *systemic space*, which contributed to both understanding the problem in terms of the family context and creating significant relationships with his parents and teacher. This motivated all the adults who interacted with Maor to be accountable for his journey. His teacher's and parents' genuine acceptance served as a lever to instill change in their understanding of Maor and in directing him towards changes in his life.

The personal space is significant in every therapeutic process and is essential when dealing with aggression due to the many challenges the therapist faces when trying to contain the client in cases where there is an aggressive threat to the therapeutic process and room. Drawing helped me to identify with Maor's story, understand the traps that could sabotage the process and avoid them for Maor's sake.

In all these spaces, the application of the dialectic principle can offer *acceptance*, empathy and a meaningful relationship, along with the commitment to *change*. It is worth noting that the case study of Maor is in fact a composite derived from the cases I and others have experienced. Maor is a figment of my imagination and yet parts of him exist in every one of us or at least in the hearts of our clients.

Acknowledgments

I would like to thank the art therapists Frida Lifshitz, Revital Turiski and Sorina Bieber for their contribution to some of the examples cited in this chapter.

References

Lahad, M. (2000a). *Creative supervision*. London: Jessica Kingsley.

Mann, J. (1973). *Time-limited psychotherapy*. Cambridge, MA: Harvard University Press.

Nissimov-Nahum, E. (2007). *The experiences, perceptions and practices of art therapists in the treatment of aggressive children in educational settings* (Ph.D dissertation). UK, University of Sussex.

Nissimov-Nahum, E. (2008). A model for art therapy in educational settings with children who behave aggressively. *The Arts in Psychotherapy*, *35*, 341–348.

Nissimov-Nahum, E. (2009). Use of a drawing task to study art therapists' personal experiences in treating aggressive children. *The Arts in Psychotherapy*, *36*, 140–147.

Nissimov-Nahum, E. (2013). *Colours of soul and mind: Art therapy for children who behave aggressively*. Tel-Aviv: Mofet. (Hebrew).

Prochaska, J.O., Norcross, J.C., & DiClemente, C.C. (1994). *Changing for Good*. New York: Morrow.

9 ECRAB (An Emotional, Cognitive, Rehabilitative and Behavioral Model)

Group-class Arts Therapy in a Special Education School

Mickey Ofer-Yarom, Deborah Court and Adina Shamir

Introduction

Arts therapists working in the educational system are called upon to deal with crucial ethical and professional issues arising from the underlying differences in approaches of professions that are often defined as distinct "professional cultures" (Moriya, 2006; Wengrower, 2001). However, given the many benefits and accomplishments of multidisciplinary teamwork, genuine serious efforts are being made to bridge these differences in schools and pre-schools (Nissimov-Nahum, 2008). This chapter discusses research (Ofer-Yarom, 2014) that has empirically examined the contribution and significance of collaborative work between arts therapists and educational teams in a group-class arts therapy setting.

The Emotional, Cognitive, Rehabilitative and Behavioral (ECRAB) model presented in this chapter applies to arts therapy in a group setting where an arts therapist is the facilitator for a group that meets at the set time allotted by the class schedule in special education schools. The classroom teacher, the assistant and all the students are present during these sessions which are held each week. The arts therapist works with the classroom staff to lead creative and experiential activities involving different art media ranging from visual art, drama, dance/movement, music to written texts. The arts therapist and the classroom staff observe the students' artwork, respond to the creative work and to other content that emerges during the creative process and encourage dialogue between students. At the end of the hour-long session, the arts therapist, the teacher and the assistant meet to discuss the session, the implications for the students and processes that tend to re-occur in the classroom.

In Israel, the concept of group-class arts therapy in special education classrooms was developed by Nissimov-Nahum (1999). Her work serves as the basis for this model, which is also guided by three basic assumptions that draw on group therapy theory (Bion, 1961), group therapy for children (Shechtman, 2010) and group therapy for children with special needs (Thompson & Trice-Black, 2012). The first is that group therapy with students from the same class, with all that this implies, can help each student progress in terms of social, behavioral and cognitive functioning within the class as a group which learns and operates socially and behaviorally within the school framework. The second is that the presence and integration of the classroom teachers and assistants in these is crucial to both the educational staff and the students because it contributes to the processes that take place during therapy and enables teachers and staff to identify and distill information and processes that occur "in real time." The third is that a combination of therapeutic approaches (ECRAB) provides an optimal therapeutic method to generate long-term effective outcomes. The model presented below reflects changes in the model resulting from research based on Nissimov-Nahum's (1999) theory and other theoretical assumptions.

Theoretical Background

The political, social and moral perceptions of society with regard to people with disabilities have influenced the development of special education frameworks and led to a worldview that authorizes people with disabilities to be allowed freedom of choice to participate in decisions related to the pursuit of their goals for self-realization in their personal lives, even if their behavior is inconsistent with social norms, and codifies the demand that institutions treat them with respect (Bank-Mikkelsen, 1980; Nirje, 1985; Wolfensberger, 1972). The implementation of a humanist worldview (Maslow & Mittelmann, 1941; Rogers, 1951, 1961, 1980) in special education settings seeks to treat the healthy parts of the student's personality as a focal point for education and development. This perception has led to the integration of paramedical services in the special education system, which includes arts therapies. The ECRAB model is used by arts therapists who implement emotional, cognitive, rehabilitative and behavioral therapeutic approaches.

The Emotional Approach

The emotional approach in education is based on a humanistic philosophy whose central figures – Dewey, Maslow, Rogers, Pereira and others – believed that people were "created in God's image" and naturally aspire towards goodness. Therefore, in an atmosphere of freedom, love and acceptance, they can exhibit the positive qualities inherent in them. In this sense, the process is more important than the result, because a person is constantly evolving and never becomes a finished product. The arts therapies adhere to these principles. Another major tenet is the belief that the arts are therapeutic forms of expression that engage the client from the start of the work process. The focus of arts therapies is an understanding of art images and products. The interpretation of artworks constitutes the essence of the depth of communication in art therapies. This implies that for a child or adult client, the arts can serve as alternate means of communication independent of spoken language (Case & Dalley, 1990). The integration of the educational-humanist philosophy, together with the notion that artwork is a central focus of therapy, govern its implementation in the education system.

In group arts therapies, as with any group process, conscious and unconscious relationships are formed between the individual's relationship with the self and with other members of the group (Bion, 1961). Group therapy allows for the examination of the client's relationship with the peer group and with internalized authority figures (such as parents) and real authoritative figures (teachers, administrators and managers at a later age; Foulkes & Anthony, 1965). Group arts therapies sessions focus on the triangular relationship between the client, the therapist and the artwork (Malchiodi, 1999; Nissimov-Nahum, 2008) and allow for intuitive and spontaneous activities through which clients can gain an awareness of subjects and aspects of their personality that they were previously unaware of and which the verbal process has failed to address. The artwork in and of itself is therapeutic and when it functions within a group setting, it inspires individuals to engage in creativity, encourages mutual assistance and positive social action. The advantage of group arts therapies lies in its ability to help individuals feel comfortable with themselves and provide them with a pleasant and often uplifting experience through their sense of belonging to the group, their sense of achievement in creating an artwork and the mutual contribution of acceptance (Yalom & Leszcz, 2005).

Group arts therapies facilitate emotional processing and focus on the relationship between the students and their peers and the educational staff while attempting to create an understanding and empathetic environment where personalities can evolve and grow in a healthy way. This approach emphasizes the warm and caring sentiments that should form the basis of the teacher-student relationship, their dialogue, their mutual openness to ideas and the sincerity guiding their relationship.

The Cognitive Approach

The cognitive approach emerged in the United States in the 1950s as an extension of the principles of the behavioral approach. It considers that an individual's thoughts reflect his/her interpretation of an event and not the event itself. This approach is based on the assumption that the individual's patterns of thinking influence his/her behavior, and that distorted thinking patterns cause emotional disorders. Cognitive therapy focuses on identifying problematic thinking patterns and replacing them with more adaptive patterns (Essar, Palgi, Ronen, & Ben-Ezra, 2010).

The cognitive approach is based on the idea that individuals' understanding of their emotions and the emotions of others can help them function appropriately or even optimally. Therefore, individuals should increase their awareness of opinions, attitudes and appraisals of situations involving emotions to resolve issues as a function of this heightened awareness of emotions and their effects on thought processes. The cognitive approach is oriented towards the immediate resolution of problems (typically those problems that the client wants to address) while encouraging the client to identify them, acquire skills to deal with them and learn how to benefit from life experiences. These techniques can help a student solve interpersonal problems which are part of everyday life in school between friends and with teachers. Research shows that the cognitive approach contributes primarily to social acceptance and the ability to demonstrate self-control, both of which are areas that special education students typically struggle with (Causton-Theoharis & Malmgren, 2005).

The Rehabilitative Approach

The rehabilitative approach focuses on preparing the student for independent functioning to the greatest possible extent. The rehabilitative approach has evolved as society has changed its stances towards democracy, pluralism and multiculturalism, and is widely accepted in therapy directed towards individuals who have physical, mental, intellectual and social disabilities. The rehabilitative approach centers on the individual and not on the disability, with the aim of integrating the individual into society independently, in terms of occupational, social and everyday functioning (Melia, Pledger, & Wilson, 2003). This approach also implements social intervention programs to help raise awareness and change the attitudes of corporations, enterprises and communities (Fornes, 2013).

The rehabilitative approach is implemented in three main arenas. In the *physical arena*, rehabilitation works to improve the independent functioning of the individual through various aids/devices/techniques, methods of compensation to carry out certain activities, and in sync with the environment for the individual to function in society and in daily life. In the *cognitive arena*, rehabilitation is designed to improve cognitive processing abilities and adaptation to the environment to improve daily functioning. In the *psychosocial arena*, the primary goal of therapy is full integration into society and the improvement of quality of life of people with disabilities to live a meaningful life. Rehabilitative intervention involves a collaboration with the individual regarding the chosen goals of therapy.

The Behavioral Approach

The behavioral approach emerged about 60 years ago as an extension of the philosophy of behaviorism developed by Skinner (1974) and various principles that were formulated later. Its basic tenet is that functional and psychological difficulties can be explained in learning and information processing terms, and therefore can legitimize and account for an individual's behavior (Hazlett-Stevens & Craske, 2002). Behavior is defined as any action that the individual voluntarily performs (whether observed or reported) that affects him/her. Behavioral interventions aim to increase self-control and the ability to regulate emotions through a variety of activities to help achieve optimal developmental results.

In the behavioral approach, all human behaviors have consequences. When there is a desired consequence, it promotes and develops the individual, and when it is undesirable, it causes the individual to avoid this behavior in the future. Its related educational philosophy encourages reinforcing desired behavior rather than using punishment. The difficulties faced by the individual are considered to emerge from environmental factors and events, so that modifying the behavior of significant people in the individual's life is expected to lead to a change in behavior. In order for this to occur, information about the student's natural environment needs to be accessed to direct the client towards new learning. During the 1980s, behavioral and cognitive therapy methods were combined into what is known now as Cognitive-Behavioral Therapy (CBT) (Butler, Chapman, Forman, & Beck, 2006).

The ECRAB model incorporates these four different therapy approaches. It is used by arts therapists to create change and a meaningful process when working with children in general and particularly with students in special education settings.

Description of the Working Model

Eight arts therapists, eight teachers, eight assistants and three national supervisors in the field of art therapy were asked to describe their case studies, experiences and stories specific to group-class therapy sessions as part of a broader project conduced at Bar Ilan University (Ofer-Yarom, 2014). Semi-structured in-depth interviews were conducted to better understand working relationships and the experiences of all those who applied the ECRAB model in schools. The interviews lasted about an hour and a half and were recorded (with prior consent of the interviewees) and transcribed. The interview data were analyzed according to the principles of categorized content analysis. Participant observation was also conducted in one group-class therapy that was active throughout the entire school year, and at the concluding session of the class year, in addition to random observations in the school yard and in the teachers' room. In addition, material was gathered from photographs taken during the observations, a "researcher diary" and a "reflexive diary" written by the arts therapist, the class teacher and the assistant at the end of each therapeutic class session in which observations were carried out.

Preparing for Group Sessions in the ECRAB Model

In the ECRAB model, the work process begins during the preparation stage for the academic year. The arts therapists and the classroom staff meet just before the start of the school year for an introductory session designed to build a system of trust and rapport. Matching expectations with the educational staff involve getting to know the students through the staff's perspective, learning their preferential instructional style (focusing on games, creative work or verbal sessions) and the content that is important for classroom interventions. In addition, the arts therapists share their expectations in terms of the level of intervention-participation from the educational staff. This leads to discussions on the code of conduct in the classroom as it compares to the rules during the therapy group sessions, which includes the red lines in both settings, as well as responses to behavioral problems. This meeting is extremely important and lays the foundation for the partnership and level of trust that are crucial to the collaborative work process (Friedman, 2002). It also provides an initial introduction for the classroom teachers to the specific arts therapies' toolbox.

Time Frame

There is no straightforward answer to the question of whether working with a group for one academic year is better than working with the same group for several years. On the one hand, research shows that some students seek stability, strengthening of the relationship formed during the first year and the opportunity to make the most of the artistic medium that the therapist uses. On the other, the school system itself imposes restrictions such as changes in terms of class hours and days, the composition of the group and its needs for diversity, with different work methods. Given that there is no specific recommendation on this issue, it is advisable to discuss the issue of the therapy time frame and to listen to the preferences of the arts therapist and the educational staff.

A Fixed Hour in the Weekly Schedule

Group-class therapy needs to be an integral part of the weekly schedule. It should take place on a set day and at a set hour when the students, the teacher, the assistant and the arts therapist are all present in the classroom. During the activity, the educational staff is attentive to the process and the students' needs. The participation and intervention of the educational staff needs to mesh with the dialogue and decisions made during the preparatory discussion and training sessions throughout the year. The findings from the observations in the Bar Ilan study (Ofer-Yarom, 2014) indicate that the educational staff can "relax" during the activity, because educational responsibility is not essential during this hour. However, in the ECRAB model, the educational staff is not permitted to engage in other classroom or personal matters but be present and participate in the creative processes and observe the processes that the students experience. The goal is that the group-class hour of therapy should be an opportunity for the educational staff to observe the students and become familiar with other sides of their personalities as creators, artists, members of a social group and more generally as both individuals and part of the whole.

Training the Educational Staff

At a set time once every two weeks, the arts therapist and the educational staff take part in a training session. The purpose is to provide a platform for dialogue which can contribute to the level of communication and quality of the relationship between therapists and teachers, match their expectations, create verbal and nonverbal codes for cooperative conduct, and process events and processes that took place during the group-class therapy sessions. These training sessions also allow the educational staff to consult about specific students or processes that occur during day-to-day interactions in the classroom.

Multidisciplinary Meeting

Once every two weeks (alternating between the training sessions), a multidisciplinary team meeting is held which is attended by management staff, the teacher, the assistant, the other teachers who teach the specific class, the arts therapist and the students' personal arts therapists, in the case where they have individualized sessions (this may be the same arts therapist, not always). During this meeting, general processes in the classroom are discussed, as well as the individual progress of each student in the class. This is an opportunity for the class arts therapist to share the emotional aspects of the classroom processes with the entire educational staff.

Working with One Group

The findings suggested that facilitating more than one group-class therapy according to the ECRAB model places a significant emotional and technical burden on the arts therapist that ultimately undermines the quality of the group process and the training of the educational staff. The savings in terms of cost do not appear to be worthwhile. Rather, it is important to ensure that therapists only facilitate one group-class therapy each year, even at the expense of not offering group-class arts therapy to every class.

Should the Activity Be Held in the Arts Therapy Room or in the Classroom?

Some arts therapists prefer to hold the group-class therapy sessions in the arts therapy room in the same space where they typically have individual sessions, arguing that the different space of the arts therapy room allows students to detach themselves from classroom patterns of behavior and experience new relationships and patterns. In addition, the games and the creative materials in the arts therapy room allow therapists to use them freely and spontaneously. Other arts therapists prefer having the group-class therapy sessions in the homeroom, where the therapy hour is perceived as a direct continuation of the educational-therapeutic process that occurs throughout the day, and where important behavioral patterns for the group-class process are reconstructed in the classroom space. If group-class therapy is held in the classroom, it is advisable to change the seating arrangement to create a different space from the day-to-day classroom setting. The seating arrangement (in a circle, on a rug, working in pairs, and others) should be chosen in terms of the special needs of the students.

Clinical Examples

The central issues in the ECRAB model as well as processes that unfold gradually with the development of the group that emerged from the Ofer-Yarom study (2014) are presented below along with brief examples of exercises and activities that enable and encourage the introduction of this content into the group-class space.

Addressing the Experience of Belonging to and Being Part of the Group

Special education students often have difficulty integrating with their peers because of their emotional difficulties, such as low frustration tolerance, difficulties in self-regulation and self-expression, as well as their impaired self-image due to physical detachment from their immediate environment (placing them in special education settings). These difficulties often lead to feelings of frustration and anxiety, and behavioral expressions of these emotions interfere with their sense of belonging and social integration, even within the special education classroom. These students need assistance at a basic level, such as helping them to express their feelings and desires, as well as their higher level skills, such as understanding and considering their own feelings and desires and those of others (Causton-Theoharis & Malmgren, 2005). Thus, the central content of the group-class therapy model is geared towards building a sense of belonging and "togetherness."

Numerous exercises can be designed to foster a sense of belonging in class and "togetherness," all of which involve collaborative creative work. One example is creating a "house" from a large cardboard box. The students paint, decorate and design the "house" and select its location in the classroom. It becomes a private and joint space for them. Another example of collaborative work involves drawing, performance and shared storytelling. Here, each student draws a personal segment, places it in a larger drawing and writes a story about the segment. One group-class story can be created from these personal stories. While working on the exercise, the students experience the joy of creating, and the pleasant atmosphere strengthens the connection between them. Note that while there is a sense of enjoyment, disagreements, quarrels or differences in opinion may arise as they do in any group process. The role of the arts therapist is to conceptualize what is happening and have a discussion that can contain these experiences of disagreement and differences within the group and legitimize this situation as a developmental stage of the group process. In this way, the arts therapist clarifies and raises awareness among the group members about new meanings with respect to themselves and their relationships with others. This significant experience consists of other aspects, as described below.

Communication Skills

Analysis of the interview data suggested that due to difficulties in the development of communication skills for many special education students, skills that may be new for them need to be incorporated such as listening to each other, being considerate of each other and even being able to compliment and praise other members of the group. In the ECRAB model, during the group-class therapy hour the staff circulates among the students to hear their opinions on general issues and try to solve problems together. Listening to the opinion of each and every participant (respect), recognizing that there is room for individual opinions yet acknowledging that a decision will be made according to the needs of the majority (listening and consideration), the positive reinforcement of personal choices and finding solutions, as well as the ability to cooperate and make decisions (praise), can help to establish good communication habits. A space of attentive listening and consideration of others can encourage students as well as the educational staff to use the group-class therapy hour to resolve issues that have surfaced outside the classroom therapy hour and best deal with them during this hour.

A number of exercises can help implement communication skills. For example, each group session can start with a round of greetings of: "How are you doing?" that includes objects (a ball or a little fuzzy doll), where each member of the group speaks while holding the object in his/her hands. Another is an exercise of praise in which each student receives two notes containing two names of students in the class. Each student is asked to write down a few words to describe the student's achievement/s over the past week. Another possibility is to initiate simulations and role-playing of everyday life events in which the dramatic experience can help students distance themselves from the event and understand how their peers react in the same situation.

"A Safe Space"

The findings indicated that creating a safe, secure and empowering therapeutic environment enables the participants to acquire skills that will help them cope with distress, which is important to the students, teachers, assistants and arts therapists alike. The educational staff interviewed in the Ofer-Yarom study emphasized the need to devote both thought and actions to prevent abusive behavior among group members and to create a sense of security in the group-class therapy space. The arts therapists who took part in the study stated that the concept of a "safe space" is suggestive of building positive defenses that protect the individual. One instance is protection from the disclosure of personal information that may be used against those who are open and honest, make them feel rejected or put them in danger of exploitation (the threat of exposing personal information to those outside of the therapy group). The sense of a "safe space" is also important for the staff as it allows them to discuss more personal issues. The educational staff felt that group-class therapy served as a safe place to present complex issues to the students.

A safe space in the group can be created by producing artwork that addresses the subject of safe spaces and by identifying its characteristics for each member of the group (such as making a large "house" from cardboard as described above) and through guided imagery exercises. However, to maintain a sense of a "safe space," it is important to ensure clear and fair rules and make sure that attentive adults are present who help preserve a respectful discussion between members of groups who disagree with one another.

When and if for whatever reason an overall sense of security cannot be achieved, the possibility of expressing feelings of unstable and vulnerability is used as a form of protection, even if it is an ineffective defense. Recognizing and acknowledging the sense of insecurity in the group affirms and validates the feelings of the group members and prevents the denial of the situation and the devaluation of members of the group.

Legitimacy of Expressing Feelings

The findings suggested that ECRAB enables participants to express complex and often strong emotions in the presence of the educational staff. The ability to express these feelings apparently emerged from the close relationships formed within the group and stemmed from the sense of "togetherness," as well as the acquired communication skills and the sense of physical and emotional security shared by all participants. The involvement of the educational staff in this process created a close relationship between teachers and students, both within and outside group-class therapy sessions, provided legitimacy of the expression of feelings for students in the classroom and demonstrated to them that personal expression in a safe, protected and respectful manner is possible. For example, at the start of one of the group-class therapy sessions, a student entered when she was upset and stated: "I'm angry at the assistant." After another student told her that she might be punished if she talked that way, she replied: "I'll be angry on the inside." The assistant sensed that the student was behaving differently and encouraged her to share her feelings, thereby expressing her anger towards the assistant. This event illustrates how group-class therapy allows for the expression of difficult feelings, even when they are connected to the relationships between students and the educational staff. The narratives collected during the study indicated that the presence of the arts therapist engendered a calm atmosphere of mutual respect and a sense of security that enabled the students and the assistant to deal with the event that involved turbulent feelings and encouraged a real-time discussion. The students in the classroom who observed the process learned the "language" of dialogue management. Through structured exercises, playing and art making, the students can better express themselves and their experiences, learn about their emotions and develop empathy for others. Becoming acquainted with different emotions through the activities in the therapy group helps the students to verbally share their inner experiences with others. The arts therapist's structured therapeutic interventions encourage students to cope with intense emotional experiences, which the therapist processes and verbally "returns" to the group, allowing members to contain them. In addition, these interventions and the group processes that follow can contribute to reducing inappropriate behavior in the classroom, such as avoidance, obstinacy and aggression. The continuation and growth of the group is made possible by the arts therapist's reflections and consideration, the intervention techniques that he/she implements that promote change and the processing that he/she "submits" to the group.

The Individual as Expressing the Voice of a Group

Another facet of expressing emotions in the group-class therapy setting that emerged from the study is the individual's ability to express the voice of a group. The individuals comprise and create the "whole" which forms the group. Different theorists have described the joint group space in different ways, including as an intersubjective space (Ogden, 1994) or a wider mind (Bateson, 1979; Gilligan, 1997), which provides a broader space of identity for the individual, a space created from the group interaction between the individuals. Figure 9.1 illustrates the importance given to emotional expression during the therapy sessions. The purpose of the activity was to familiarize the students with a variety of words that describe emotions (for example, embarrassment, enjoyment, relief, jealousy) to expose the students to a rich emotional language.

The findings suggested that group-class therapy allows individuals to reveal their personal "story," feelings, conflicts and concerns in a protected space. The topics that the individual discloses belong to him/her, but they are also part of the "group voice" that emerges from the collective unconscious of the group, the intersubjective space. The topics that an individual contributes allow all the members of the group to clarify what feelings and

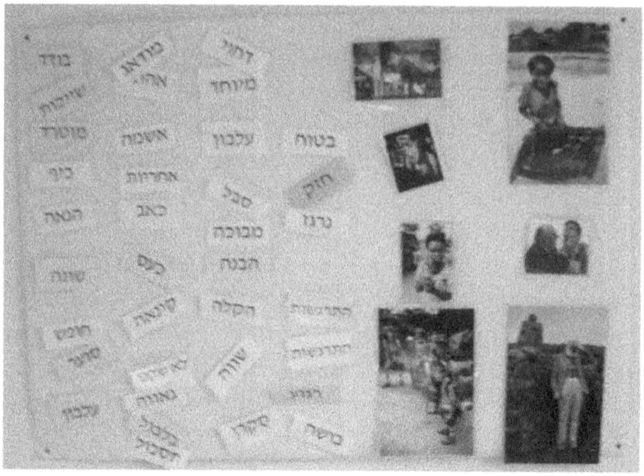

Figure 9.1 "Emotional Expression" – a Variety of Words and Pictures for Emotions – an Image Created by the Classroom Staff with the Arts Therapist and That Hangs on the Wall in the Group-class Therapy Room.

emotions are present in their own similar emotional experience. The role of the group facilitator is to develop and enrich the discussion by turning it into a group discussion that expresses the feelings of the individual and the group alike. An example of this process took place (in the discussion below) between the arts therapist and one of the students concerning problems that arose during the week. This discussion caused another student to recall a traumatic event that some of the adults in her life were trying to keep secret, and she kept it to herself until that moment:

Therapist: Now is a good time to share something that happened to you this week, something good or problematic. Yoni (student) gave me an idea because he shared a problem that he had, and how he handled it.

Avi (student): It's something not good. On Friday I got stuck in the bathroom, and Daniel (student) rescued me, he kicked in the door, and it opened.

Yael (student): Were you scared?

Avi (student): remains silent.

Therapist: Yael asked if you were afraid.

Avi: Very, they broke down the door.

Yael: He probably said to himself: Maybe, surely someone will come and rescue me. How do I know?

Therapist: Are you guessing or asking him if that's how he felt?

Yael: I didn't say anything. At my previous school, I was in the kitchen, and a girl came up to me, she was bigger than me, and turned the light off, and closed the door, and I couldn't get out. Then the girl's

> mother came and yelled at her and then my mother came and gave me a big hug.

The experience of fear as described by Avi (student) to the group created a sense of legitimacy and a universality of the fear, which was shared by the students and adults alike, thus allowing Yael (student) to speak openly about it. The group structure that served as a framework for the manifestation of processes allowed the student to "let go" of a story that was locked within and express the emotions that accompanied the experience. This was done without fear of judgment or anger, which allowed her to process her own traumatic experience.

The Meaning of the Disability for the Individual

The experiences related to the students' disabilities are often accompanied by different degrees of emotional reactions, and these experiences are likely to be expressed during the group-class therapy sessions due to their collective nature. However, the findings suggested that dealing with disabilities and the effects they have on the individual are vital and characteristic of all class therapy groups in the special education settings. For the individual, the disability also involves coping with stigmas. The educational staff interviewed in the study mentioned various aspects of the stigma that included attending school events, occasionally for the first time in their lives, their fear of the effects of medication, pressures in the family when one sibling has complex disabilities, the perception of the disability as a "contagious disease" as well as the attitudes and feelings of the professionals working with students who are diagnosed with severe and complex disabilities.

The use of literary texts and films that address either the characteristics of the disability or the stigmatization can contribute to discussions on this topic. The processing should include aspects such as: Did you happen to form an opinion about someone just because you did not know them? What did you feel? What did you think? What did you do? Has anyone ever formed an opinion about you in the same way? How did you feel? What did you think? What did you do? Did you ever change your opinion about someone after you got to know them? What did you feel? What did you think? What did you do? Thus, group-class therapy appears to give a sense of belonging and provide a social setting for special education students. Feelings of belonging and "togetherness" are the main issues that these types of groups address.

Creating and Creativity As a Therapeutic Force

Activities with different art materials and techniques form the basis for working in the arts therapies. The actual engagement in creative group work mobilizes the creative and healthy forces of the group and the individuals within it (Thompson, 2009). For this reason, ECRAB emphasizes the healing power of art (art as therapy). The creative work brings the group together and enables the establishment of values, such as collaboration and consideration, which is also achieved without verbal communication. The arts therapy room the class enters is full of creative materials (see Figures 9.2(a) and 9.2(b)) and conveys a sense of "something else," a sense of creation, creativity and self-expression. The variety of art materials allows for free expression of opinions and ideas. This is not a "regular" school classroom, but a place where students are encouraged to express themselves in different ways.

The findings suggest that working with both art materials and games increased the clients' motivation to create and perform. The use of diverse techniques and artistic images enabled a variety of expressive possibilities and highlighted the opportunities for the students to express themselves while recognizing and becoming acquainted with their environment and the skills required to integrate into it. The use of artistic-expressive materials and techniques allowed the students to think abstractly, use and expand their capacities of symbolization, and expand their cognitive abilities through the art and creative exercises. For example, before the celebration of "Tu BiShvat" (the Jewish New Year of the Trees), one of the arts therapists held a discussion in the group about making personal wishing trees during which she talked about the growth and life cycle of trees over time. The students understood the comparison between the life of a tree and the life of a human and relationship between the fruit of the tree and the fruit of the family in one's children, and thus shared their personal growth experiences with each other. The activity allowed the educational staff to get to know another side of their students' lives.

The skills set that is required of the students during the group-class therapy is different from the one needed during regular classroom lessons, and the atmosphere in the group-class therapy is different from the atmosphere in a lesson. This allows for new content and different aspects of the students' personalities to surface, as one teacher noted:

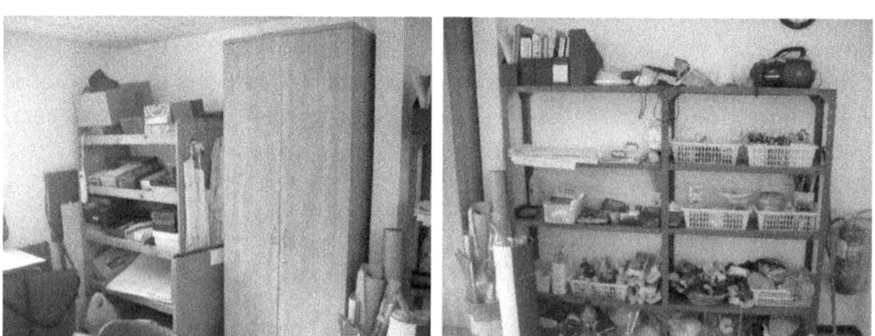

Figures 9.2(a) and 9.2(b) The Diversity of Creative Materials Conveys a Sense of Creativity.

> The opportunities to see her [the student] in another way, and to understand her emerged clearly in class therapy. We saw that during the class therapy, she took on the role of class clown. A student who studied in a regular school until eighth grade, was a shadow there.... She would walk down the corridor rubbing against the walls with her head down. Of all people, she was the one who was cheeky in the group, and we suddenly saw how much she enjoyed the reactions of the people around her. In this way, we realized what a strong need she had for social interaction, and her strengths. We might have never seen this because she does not disclose this side of her during class.

The creative work appears to have served as a "passage" between the arts therapies and the school, between the individual's "inner world" and "the outside world." Group-class therapy enabled the student's "inner world" to acquire symbolic expression (the artwork) in the presence of classmates and the educational staff while being processed, supported and contained by the arts therapist. Later in this process, the artworks can serve as a kind of transitional object (Winncott, 1971) or "self-objects" (Kuhot, 1984) for the students and provide a source of reassurance, security and pride. One of the arts therapists described an instance in which she allowed students to remove their artwork from the therapy room because she felt they had meaning for them in "real life" outside the therapy room:

> They (the students) put on a joint show for the end of year party. They took the masks that we made during the year...I don't think that it's good to take things out of the therapy room and transfer them to a different context because there is the therapeutic context. Here I felt that they were taking them and using them proudly, and it transitioned with them in their lives, and it's like there is something that flows forward.

The creative ideas that emerged and were implemented during the group-class therapy were used by the educational staff within the class framework. For example, one of the classes wrote a behavioral contract during group-class therapy. The contract, signed by the staff and the students, was hung on the classroom notice board, and served the educational staff and students throughout the week. In a different classroom, a classroom "time-out" corner was designated for rest and relaxation during the group-class therapy sessions and this was used every school day. In addition, the teachers, inspired by art and creativity, also occasionally discovered new things about themselves. For example, one teacher discovered her love of painting during the arts therapy hour.

The creative work seemed to permeate the classroom experience, and contributed significantly to "spiritual knowledge," the sensitivity and awareness of the meaning of the artwork, to decency in human interactions and to increasing the awareness of the feelings of the students and the educational staff, even outside the group therapy setting.

Relaxation Techniques

The routine of school life, for both students and the educational staff, is highly stressful. As a result, teaching mental relaxation techniques during group-class therapy is highly beneficial. During the sessions, the group continues to work on content and skills that are required of the students, but this is carried out in a relaxed atmosphere. For the students, the arts therapy session provides a break from academic pressures, and therefore allows for a relaxed atmosphere of playfulness and creativity.

Figures 9.3(a) and 9.3(b) that were photographed during a group-class arts therapy observation illustrate a type of relaxation activity. They show how the students move with fabrics while calm music is playing in the background. Various relaxation methods can be implemented such as flexing and releasing different parts of the body, warming the hands by rubbing them together and massaging each other's shoulders in pairs or behind one another in a circle.

If the arts therapist chooses to work in the therapy room, the change will start with the difference in setting from the classroom. The curtains, the large armchairs and the carpet create a different atmosphere and convey a feeling that "rest is allowed in this place." Some arts therapists in the study used these techniques during group-class therapy or as part of the educational staff training to promote personal and group processes. Avinon (2000) mentioned the relaxation and "recharging" elements that embody creativity and playfulness for teachers. He noted that combining play and relaxation without the fear of loss of control or attention allows for a space to address different phenomena that emerge from rigidity and burnout, and are important for promoting values such as openness and sensitivity

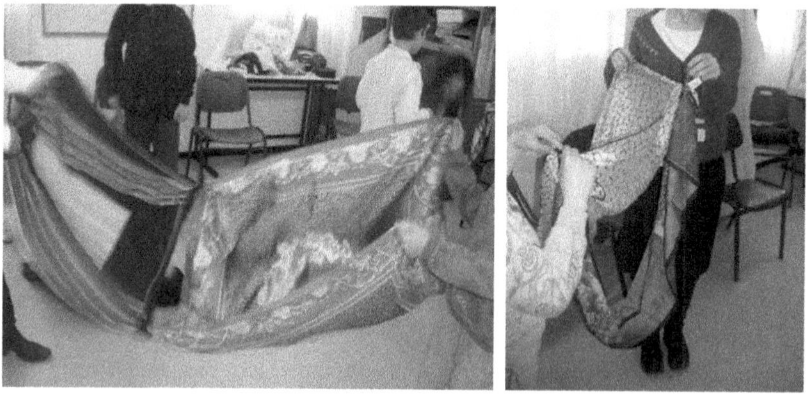

Figures 9.3(a) and 9.3(b) Activity Involving Moving with Fabrics and Quiet Music.

to perspectives on concepts such as good and bad, beautiful and ugly, and true and false.

In the ECRAB, consideration of the needs of the individual and the group, the encouragement of emotional expression, the atmosphere of freedom of thought and expression, the sense of comfort, and the containment and absence of judgmental attitudes all merge together to produce a safe and protective space for individuals and the group. Relaxation that occurs within a framework where the client feels protected enables therapeutic processes to emerge and generates behavioral change within the group interaction (Shechtman, 2010). Setting appropriate boundaries helps both students and staff members avoid improper content and offensive behavior or statements, and in doing so, students learn to protect themselves and use resources in a way that fits their needs. The ultimate goal is to gradually transfer the responsibility for setting desired boundaries for optimal social functioning to the students.

This combination of feelings of relaxation and preserving boundaries emerged clearly in one class. In all of the sessions, the arts therapist used a white cloth to cover a closet full of games that the students could not access during the group-class therapy (see Figure 9.4). This conveyed a clear message to the students that not everything is permitted in the room and there are specific things that they are not allowed to do, and that the surroundings (the room) is designed to correspond to the students' abilities, difficulties and needs. One of the goals of covering the closet and the games was to make it easier for students who struggle to concentrate on the group task because they want to play.

On a more general level, this example illustrates the extent to which the arts therapists continued to think about the needs of the students, gave them

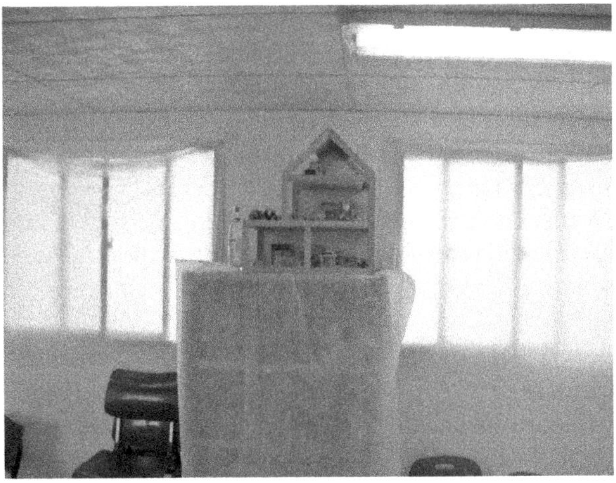

Figure 9.4 The Covered Games Closet.

a sense that they were visible and made room for their wishes at the right time, as underscored in Kohut's Self Psychology (Kohut, 1984). In addition, the therapists also try to protect the educational staff by allowing them to express themselves emotionally while maintaining their privacy as adults while adjusting the content to the setting with the students. The training of the arts therapists to accept different behaviors in an empathetic and patient manner while protecting themselves and the students is important and aids in the processes presented above. The message is that the needs of the individual must be taken into account while considering the needs of the rest of the group and day to day reality. Besides the conversations about the participants' emotional sides, a dialogue also takes place about maintaining physical health and awareness of the students' personal safety.

Summary and Conclusions

The purpose of this chapter was to describe the ECRAB group-class therapy model that includes the classroom educational team (teachers and assistants). The foundation and origins of this work are based on humanistic education approaches and principles, and innovative educational perceptions that aspire towards the best possible collaboration between the various bodies working within the school for the benefit of the student and the entire system, as well as the insights and principles of arts therapies and cognitive, rehabilitative and behavioral therapies.

In the model, the basis of the process during group-class therapy involves the use of the art materials as healing agents as well as the ability to combine relaxation and a sense of release (both physically and mentally) while maintaining a setting that is secure and governed by rules. The use of art materials and art making in general help to address a diverse range of issues, contributes to developing social and communication skills, fosters decency in human relations and raises awareness of the feelings of both students and educational staff outside of the therapeutic group setting. The relaxation incorporated into the sessions allows for emotional release and comfort without harming others. The relaxation techniques take the needs of others, the classroom rules that protect everyone, and the safeguard of the body and possessions into account. When this integration is embedded within the school, an environment is created that is focused on the individual while taking the system into consideration. This type of environment can scaffold growth of the mind, and in particular the development of special education students.

References

Avinon, J. (2000). *Goals and values in education*. Kiryat Biyalick: Aach Pbulishing. (in Hebrew).

Bank-Mikkelsen, N.E. (1980). Denamrk. In R.J. Flynn, & K.E. Nitsch (Eds.), *Normalization, social integration and community services* (pp. 51–70). Baltimore: University Park Press.

Bateson, G. (1979). *Mind and nature: A necessary unity*. Cresskill, NJ: Hampton Press.

Bion, W.R. (1961). *Experiences in groups*. London: Tavistock.

Butler, A.C., Chapman, J.E., Forman, E.M., & Beck, A.T. (2006). The empirical status of cognitive-behavioral therapy: A review of meta-analyses. *Clinical Psychology Review, 26*, 17–31.

Case, C., & Dalley, T. (1990). *Working with children in art therapy*. London: Routledge.

Causton-Theoharis, J.N., & Malmgren, K.W. (2005). Building bridges: Strategies to help paraprofessionals promote peer interaction. *Teaching Exceptional Children, 37*(6), 18–24.

Essar, N., Palgi, Y., Ronen, S., & Ben-Ezra, M. (2010). Pre-traumatic vaccination intervention: Can dissociate symptoms be reduced? *Pre-hospital disaster Medicine, 25*, 278–284

Fornes, S.L. (2013). *Integrating individuals with developmental disabilities into the open labor market*. USA: Florida International University.

Foulkes, S.H., & Anthony, E.J. (1965). *Group psychotherapy: The psychoanalytic approach* (2nd ed.). London: Penguin Books.

Friedman, R. (2002). Developing partnership promotes peace: Group psychotherapy experiences. *Croatian Medical Journal, 43*(2), 141–147.

Gilligan, S.G. (1997). *The courage to love: Practice and principles of self-relations psychotherapy*. New York: Norton.

Hazlett-Stevens, H., & Craske, M.G. (2002). Brief cognitive-behavioral therapy: definition and scientific foundations. In F.W. Bond, & W. Dryden (Eds.), *Handbook of brief cognitive behavior therapy* (pp. 1–20). New York: Chichester: Wiley.

Kohut, H, (1984). *How does analysis cure?* Chicago: University of Chicago Press.

Malchiodi, C.A. (1999). *Medical art therapy with children*. London: Jessica Kingsley Publishers.

Maslow, A., & Mittelmann, B. (1941). *Principles of abnormal psychology*. New York: Harper & Row.

Melia, R.P., Pledger, C., & Wilson, R. (2003). Disability and rehabilitation research: Opportunities for participation, collaboration, and extramural funding for psychologists. *American Psychologist, 58*(4), 285–288.

Moriya, D. (2006). Ethical issues in school art therapy. *Art Therapy: Journal of the American Art Therapy Association, 23*(3), 59–65.

Nirje, B. (1985). The basis and logic of the normalization principle. *Australia & New Zealand Journal of Developmental Disabilities, 11*, 65–68.

Nissimov-Nahum, E. (1999). Integrating therapeutic approaches into the art therapist's work according to a model developed at Erezim School, Rishon LeZion. *Issues in Special Education & Inclusion, 14*, 103–199. (in Hebrew).

Nissimov-Nahum, E. (2008). A model for art therapy in educational settings with children who behave aggressively. *The Arts in Psychotherapy, 35*, 341–348.

Ofer-Yarom, M. (2014). *Co-therapy by an educator and a therapist for group art-therapy within a school*. (Ph.D. Thesis, Submitted to the Senate of Bar-Ilan University), Ramat-Gan (in Hebrew).

Ogden, T.H. (1994). The analytic third: Working with intersubjective clinical facts. *International Journal of Psychoanalysis, 75*, 3–20.

Rogers, C.R. (1951). *Client-center therapy*. Boston: Houghton Mifflin.

Rogers, C.R. (1961). *On becoming a person*. Boston: Houghton Mifflin.

Rogers, C.R. (1980). *A way of being*. Boston: Houghton Mifflin.

Shechtman, Z. (2010). *Group counseling and psychotherapy with children and adolescents*. Emek Yisrael: Academic press (in Hebrew).

Skinner, B.F. (1974). *About behaviorism*. New York: Knopf.

Thompson, B. (2009). Artistic sensibility in the studio and gallery model: Revisiting process and product. *Art Therapy: Journal of the American Art Therapy Association*, *26*(4), 159–166.

Thompson, E.H., & Trice-Black, S. (2012). School-based group interventions for children exposed to domestic violence. *Journal of Family Violence*, *27*, 233–241.

Wengrower, H. (2001). Art therapies in educational settings: An intercultural encounter. *The Arts in Psychotherapy*, *28*, 109–115.

Winnicott, D.W. (1971). *Playing and reality*. Routledge, London.

Wolfensberger, W. (1972). *The principle of normalization in human services*. Toronto: National Institute on Mental Retardation.

Yalom, I.D., & Leszcz, M. (2005). *The theory and practice of group psychotherapy* (5th ed.). New York: Basic Books.

10 Dialogue through the Exhibition of Artworks

Anat Liban

Introduction

Exhibiting clients' artworks in their school setting is often considered a way to provide support to these students. This chapter addresses the ethical issues involved in exhibiting artworks, describes the preparation process and analyzes the impact on the student of exhibiting artworks to family, friends as well as the educational and therapeutic staff. Over the past four years, I have been working with my clients on exhibits of their paintings, sculptures and photographs on school grounds. In a structured and protected manner, these types of exhibitions allow clients to share their artwork that expresses their abilities to create something out of chaos, confusion, anxiety and aggression, and constitute a meaningful, sublimative and adaptive personal product. These exhibitions not only fulfill the need for visibility and validation of the subjective experience, or "the function of the inner witness" as Dana Amir (2013) terms it, but also the clients' sense of ability, competence and creativity.

The idea of setting up exhibitions emerged and developed from requests by many clients to show their artworks to their teachers, parents and classmates. This primarily captured the need to share their sense of liveliness and creativity, health and authenticity that they discovered in the art therapy room with others. I realized that a structured therapeutic process in which some of the artistic products were displayed could prepare them for this kind of exposure and help them feel that they were both seen and protected.

Theoretical Background

Presenting Clients' Artworks

In Chambala's (2008) article "Anxiety and art therapy: Treatment in the public eye," a group art therapy process is described where the artworks are presented to the public at the treatment center and in a private gallery at the university. She states that the artworks were a living testimony to the feelings, insights and thoughts of the clients and could be harnessed as an emotional-educational tool for the general public. The exhibition, which presented theoretical and research material on the subject, created a powerful experience that depicted the complexity and personal difficulties associated with various anxiety disorders. Through the display of their artworks, the clients felt that sharing their personal knowledge about the nature of the anxiety disorder enabled them to be better appreciated and understood by the general public. The opportunity to disclose meaningful experiences, demonstrate their skills and strengths, and even engender a sense of security and protection within the group who presented their artworks together has also been described by other therapists (e.g., Leenstra, Goldstraw, & Rumbold, 2014).

Although they take place in the school space, the art exhibitions set up by clients towards the end of the academic year allow them to share the inner images that form part of their art therapy processes with other people who are close to them (parents, siblings, teachers, friends). The presence of the artwork in the school space provides the clients with a sense of achievement and self-worth. In my opinion it is important that there will be many "significant others" (especially in the educational team) in attendance who will provide a curious and interested perspective for the clients. Public displays in the school also enable these students to have their expressive and creative sides recognized and admired and can contribute to meaningful change in the way they perceive themselves. It is not only important how the clients experience themselves, but also how they believe that others in their environment perceive them. This is critical and influences these students' standing in the school both socially and academically. Thus, harnessing support from parents, the educational staff and the social milieu for the therapeutic process is vital.

The importance of this process takes on particular significance in that it permits an intersection between the educational and therapeutic languages through the integration of arts therapies into schools. As an art therapist working within a systemic approach, I am aware of the tension between teachers and arts therapists. Teachers most often only encounter aggression and anxiety and its impact on the classroom, whereas the arts therapist, who is with the client in an intimate and empowering therapy room, has greater access to the client's wishes and hopes for a good and containing relationship. Exhibiting artworks in the school space is a way to bridge this gap.

Zehava Osterville (1995) discusses the need to combine two approaches that initially appear unrelated; namely, the integration of psychoanalysis with the systemic approach. According to Osterville:

> The inner world of the individual is significantly influenced by the relationship with significant figures in past and present life. Therapeutic rules for understanding the individual allow the therapist to consider, in addition to the child's emotional needs, those of the significant others in the client's life (parents and other children). The therapist

> attending to the emotional needs of the significant others in the child's life assists in mobilizing the environment for the child's benefit and promoting the restoration of a healthy developmental path.
>
> (p. 13)

Throughout my years working for the Ministry of Education, I was aware of the gap between the art therapist's perception and the educational staff's perception of the client; however, I did not appreciate the extent of the disparity. Statements such as: "Did he really do this? Who took this picture? Did he choose the title of the artwork himself? Did they work together?" clearly pointed to the need to create a bridge between my work and that of the teachers, the counselor and even the school principal.

Meeting with the parents of my clients in the exhibition space presents another opportunity to observe the different ways that the parents relate to the artworks and makes it possible to witness their authentic responses to their children's work and effort. Parents and teachers acquire greater empathy and emotional understanding of the degree of complexity, depth and emotional strength experienced by their children and students. An exhibition becomes a way to become acquainted with facets of the student that were concealed or not detected. Getting to know these sides of the student allows the professional team to gain new insights and shapes new forms of dialogue with them. The parents can benefit from a novel perspective while seeing these inner images in an empathetic, new and different way.

In an article by Osnat Weinfeld Yehudian (2013), she discusses the violation of the intimacy of the setting. She writes that in an open space, the child also engages in maintaining the imaginary walls of the therapeutic space. In this situation, the therapist and the client are jointly responsible for creating and maintaining the therapeutic environment. This also applies to the work of arts therapists in schools. The situation in which the imaginary walls of art therapy are penetrated by the educational staff is a familiar one, but the formation of the therapeutic relationship, the establishment of trust and the creation of the intermediate space in therapy help maintain the therapeutic space based on the therapeutic gaze, body language and words. The exhibitions that take place at the end of the academic year, at a time when the therapeutic relationship has been established and strengthened, authorizes a departure from the closed therapeutic space and the entry into the school space that takes into account not only the clients' difficulties, but also their emotional abilities and strengths to maintain the intermediate space.

This process often generates frustration and distressing encounters between the external and internal "realities" and allows for conflicting content that had been repressed and projected to be articulated and exposed. Exhibitions also provide a window on parts of the self that clients do not always allow therapists to reach, such as their relationships with parents, teachers, their therapy group members and classmates. This emotional content can be processed in the art therapy room after the exhibition.

Exhibitions allow for visibility, reduce the use of rigid defenses, deepen insights and lessen the intensity of anxiety and splitting, thus leading to possible growth and change. The exhibitions I set up with my clients have helped me foster and deepen relationships not only with my clients' parents, but also with the educational staff and further strengthened the systemic discourse with the school administrative staff. This chapter addresses the question of professional ethics and the description of the various work stages in which I focus on different components of my work.

Issues Related to Professional Ethics

The exhibition of clients' artworks takes place in various settings, including in mental health institutions. The ethical dilemmas surrounding exhibitions of this kind elicit extreme differences of opinion. These stem from the tradeoff between the advantages, as described above, and the risks. The concerns mentioned in the literature primarily address the impact of transferring the artwork from the therapeutic context, where there is a shared understanding between the art therapist and the client about its meaning, to the public space where they are exposed to various interpretations, some of which may influence the client creator (Leenstra et al., 2014). Other authors have discussed the clients' right to freely choose to participate in an exhibition without fearing that the therapeutic process will be terminated if they refuse to do so (Johnson, 2013).

Rand (2011), in reference to the *Ethical Principles for Art Therapists* published by the American Art Therapy Association, argued that art therapists should weigh the potential benefits of an exhibition against the drawbacks of exposing clients' work. In his view, the role of the art therapist is to protect the client from potential exploitation and abuse deriving from a public display. Johnson (2013) emphasized the need for art therapists to talk to their clients about how their work will be presented, and to assess their willingness to reveal their names and prepare the text accompanying the artworks. This conversation can help clients become aware and perhaps more fully process the meaning of their decision in the context of personal goals. Leenstra and colleagues (2014) suggested that this process should ideally take place while supporting client independence and a sense of empowerment and by focusing on notions of growth and understanding of dependency relationships. All authors cite the importance of obtaining informed consent, both from the clients who created the artworks and their legal guardians.

The key questions related to exhibitions of clients' artwork in the school space can be formulated as follows:

- Is the request to show artwork a need or a desire?
- By displaying their artwork, do clients want witnesses to their very existence, not just the physical existence of daily life, but also the more emotional and hidden parts at the core of their internal conflict?

- Does the request to present artworks originate from the feeling that others do not know they have healthy, creative and adaptive sides that need to be acknowledged?
- Does the art therapist's interest in setting up an exhibition genuinely take into account the benefits for the clients, given the clients' feelings, vulnerabilities and desires and how the exhibition can empower them?
- What can be learned from art therapists' need to present and proclaim the success of their clients in public even at the expense of violating these clients' privacy?
- What is the solution to art therapists' eternal dilemma between the need to provide visibility and empowerment and their role in maintaining the clients' privacy and shielding their vulnerability?
- Is it possible to have an exhibition in an open space and still provide a protected and safe space for these students?

In addition to these questions, there are more specific ones related to the nature of the relationship between art therapists and the educational staff in the public education system. When part of a Ministry of Education setting, arts therapists are challenged to examine, adapt and extend their therapeutic approaches.

My personal contention is that it is imperative to take advantage of all educational and school affordances to promote clients' well-being. This constitutes a shift from the clinical model of a therapist and client in a closed room towards an open therapeutic-creative approach, and community and social work. In the internal conflict between maintaining the setting and therapeutic principles and the need to change and break through the framework and integrate other interventions and therapeutic approaches that call for changing patterns, I tend to explore additional options for therapeutic approaches.

Govrin (2013) discussed this change in mindset through a socioanthropological analysis of psychoanalytic communities. He argued that a "disenchanted community" breaks the conventional frame of thought. This is characterized by dissatisfaction and an appeal for change. In contrast, "fascinated communities" do not always allow content renewal and occasionally sanction those who deviate. For example, the change in the therapeutic technique and my call for incorporating therapeutic approaches and other techniques in art therapy in the school space was not accepted by my colleagues at first. However, as the idea and working model evolved, there was a greater readiness to listen and examine the potential of the exhibition as a therapeutic tool.

Description of the Working Model and Clinical Examples

This section describes the stages of setting up the exhibition using examples from recent years of exhibitions I have held with my clients.

Stage One – selecting a Theme for the Exhibition – integrating the Educational Agenda

The first stage of the exhibition is the selection of a theme. The subject and content of the exhibitions described below emerged during the year from the artistic work in the art therapy room and from the feelings that I had throughout the school year.

First year: "Home for dreams." In the first year, many "houses" were built from cardboard cartons that we were supplied by the school maintenance man. I decided that in the exhibition we would primarily exhibit houses, so I called it "Home for dreams." I consulted with the school principal, the counselor and the students. The school maintenance man who helped us find the materials was also invited to the exhibition. He showed that he indeed connected with the intertwining of reality and imagination in the exhibition by asking if he could rent the house one of the students built.

Second year: "A recycling session." The second exhibition was called "A recycling session" and the theme of the exhibition became part of the school theme more generally. The school where I work has addressed the issues of ecology, recycling and sustainability over the years and was recently awarded the title of "Evergreen School." This direct tie between school activities and educational content prompted me to choose this theme for the exhibition. For the educational staff who teach sustainability, the exhibition took on real relevance and strengthened the commonalities of the educational and therapeutic worlds through the shared content and the ecological messages conveyed to the students in therapy. This helped eliminate the mysterious and unrelated aura surrounding the work of the art therapist and served to integrate art therapy into the educational and social system through the overarching aim of fostering clients' well-being in all areas and through collaboration with other educational actors.

Third year: "The toy symphony." In the third year, we worked with broken toys which were collected by the entire educational team and the clients for the exhibition. The idea of recruiting teachers starting from the preparation stage fascinated me because I believe that the involvement of the educational team has intrinsic value. The exhibition was called "The toy symphony." During the preparation stage, the music teacher told me that during the year the students had studied "The toy symphony" and we decided that recordings of this well-known symphony would be played in the background during the exhibition. At the exhibition I talked to the students about the many creative connections and combinations between the plastic arts and music.

The repeated use of discarded and thrown-away materials in the art therapy room is part of the school's agenda of sustainability but is also consistent with therapeutic processes where the client "creates things out of internal chaos." Winnicott (1984) argued that being able to destroy and acknowledge the destructive parts inside each individual are highly significant to emotional development and are vital to building and creating something that is valuable within the individual. Certainly at a deeper level, the "discarded, forgotten, and thrown away" raw materials were used by clients to engage in the repair and healing process by employing them in a thematic context that cannot "be destroyed," thus allowing them to experience growth, development and change.

Involving as many teachers as possible in the process created a sense of emotional engagement and solidarity and a message that the therapeutic team together with the educational team had the best interests of the students at heart and were working together towards their progress and development both emotionally and academically. This approach diminished the students' use of ineffective defense mechanisms and splitting, and thus enabled a deeper dialogue with the teachers about clients in therapy.

Fourth year: "Seeing eye to eye." In the fourth year, I decided to add photography as a technique. Photography allowed the students to avoid self-criticizing their "drawing abilities," which often arises in the art therapy room and is an obstacle to growth for some clients. The school principal allocated a considerable budget for the photographs in the exhibit, which for me was an important signal of support, involvement and sense of trust in the therapeutic process. Many of the photographs featured in this exhibition were taken in the ecological garden, another project that was created by students with the science teacher. Presenting them in the exhibition provided further concrete indications of the students' involvement in the gardening project (a significant learning process) which took place at the school.

Over the years there have been changes to the original model and perceptions of art therapy at school that express the growing partnership and involvement between myself and the educational staff. Art therapy in the educational system has thus exited the art therapy room and expanded and adjusted to the "intermediate space" where creative and therapeutic work coexist.

Stage Two – initial Preparations – exploring the Inner World

In the second stage of the preparation for the exhibition and after selecting the topic, the students meet to discuss the theme, its significance for them and how they relate to it. Preparation for the exhibition was held in the art therapy room. At this stage several questions are raised each year. First, I ask the students whether they want to present at the exhibition. The students can exhibit a selected work in the exhibition, exhibit a work anonymously or not exhibit at all. This conversation tends to elicit significant therapeutic material, which often focuses on the need to be seen, issues of self-confidence, personal and social self-image, and internal and external criticism. The clarification of these significant issues was made possible by discussing the exhibition. We think and speak aloud and finally examine the advantages and disadvantages of each alternative.

The next issue, for those students who decided to participate, is which piece of artwork should be displayed. Which ones are suitable for the exhibition? Which should not be taken from the art therapy room and into the school space (private, public, personal, interior and exterior)? Each of these raises associated questions: Why was this artwork chosen, what does it represent? What are the expectations, wishes and emotional needs? These many questions that arise during conversations with clients at various levels of depth and emotional connection provide an opportunity to expand and explore the clients' inner worlds. For example, as part of the preparation for the photography exhibition, I asked Lilac (pseudonym) some questions about the photograph she chose to present. Lilac began to wiggle uneasily in her chair. I said to her: "I see that you're not calm, maybe you'd like to tell me something? Ask me a question?" Lilac: "Yes, will our conversation about the photograph also be part of the exhibition?" I smiled and said it seemed to me that the conversation was very personal, and in the exhibition, we would only display the photograph that she would choose with its title, just as we agreed. Lilac: "Yes, I remember now." The conversation had an intimate nature and to Lilac, who tended to interpret intimacy as intrusive, this exposure aroused fear and threat. The process we went through that year was gradual and progressed at her own pace. Displaying a photograph in the exhibition exacerbated her fear of the penetrating gaze. Lilac said she wanted her siblings and parents to attend the exhibition and that she was thinking of giving the photograph to her sister as a gift. This conversation allowed me to see the progress that Lilac had made during the year, but it also served as an important reminder of the caution that I needed to maintain throughout the process.

Stage Three – Setting Up the Exhibition – Involving the Parents and Educational Staff in the Process

During the setup stage, approximately two weeks before the exhibition opens, I assign roles according to the abilities of each of my clients. The tasks include choosing a name for the exhibition, creating the invitations and distributing them, organizing and cleaning the exhibition space, taking the selected artworks to the space, arranging the exhibition and preparing a poster bearing the title of the exhibition, etc. The work is carried out collaboratively while thinking about shared responsibilities, which is an important therapeutic goal for clients who often fail to take responsibility or engage in teamwork at home or in the classroom. I make preparations with each individual client, dyad and group during the therapeutic hour assigned to them in the system. I also hold several meetings and make phone calls to the students' parents where I give them information about the preparation, the selection process and the emotional significance of the artworks that are going to be displayed. I explain the importance of their attendance for their children and talk to them about the importance of the artworks and the process. I also talk to the clients' teachers and explain the importance of classmates' reactions for the clients. I emphasize the contribution of classmates' respectful responses on the clients' self-image. In addition, I advise teachers to have a short talk about the exhibition with their students in preparation for the opening. Due to the considerable effort invested in the exhibition, it is an opportunity for classmates to get to know their friends in a different way.

For example, this year Ron's father helped us set up and prepare for the exhibition. I had worked with Ron's father throughout the year as part of the parent-child therapeutic process. Ron is a student who has been diagnosed on the autistic spectrum and is enrolled in a regular first-grade class. His father got involved in the preparation process for the exhibition together with Ron. From Ron's perspective, all changes are difficult and intimidating, and especially any deviation from the familiar therapeutic setting. However, along with his father, we were able to engage and encourage him to help cover the library shelves with sheeting and arrange the tables in the exhibition room. I sensed that Ron's father also needed to be involved in the preparations for the exhibition. His son's ability to adapt to change and deal with it not only allowed him to see how Ron had progressed during the year, but also allowed him to feel calmer and more confident that Ron could face and even overcome the difficulty and challenges he was asked to accomplish. There is no doubt that his ability to take part in the entire work process, and in each of its stages, reflected his progress but also the significance and quality of the relationship that he had established with his father throughout the year. When his classmates were invited to attend the exhibition, the task became relatively easy and feasible for him, owing mainly to his father's presence. Their relationship deepened and developed throughout the year, and their shared experience throughout the process helped Ron to prepare himself emotionally to stand in front of all the members of his class and present the artwork he had chosen.

Stage Four – the Exhibition as a Mediator

The exhibitions took place in the school library, a space that can be secured during the week after the planned visits to the exhibition. It is very important to create a space that offers a sense of security and protects the clients' artworks during the week when they are on display.

The clients' parents and family members were also invited to the exhibitions at the school. The exhibitions were held on Fridays, a day when most parents are available to come to the school and attend the exhibition, as well as the teachers and the clients' classmates. At first, the students were asked to view a presentation about the theme of the exhibition in terms of the art world. I presented several artworks by artists that addressed the themes of the exhibitions (home, ecology, recycling, photography). Then, I briefly explained the rules of conduct in the exhibition space. For example, visitors were allowed to observe, look and ask questions but not touch or photograph the artworks. For many students at the school, this was their first visit to an art exhibition.

Each client, after a visit by his/her parents and family members, presented the artworks orally. The client began by describing the use of the various materials, the work process and finally talked about the artwork. If presenting the work was challenging for the client, I asked guiding questions. Almost every time, the teachers added questions that showed their sincere interest and insights arising from their familiarity with the students, and offered words of praise and encouragement. At the end, the students could ask further questions and relate to the artworks on display. Importantly, in the exhibition space, classmates were considerate and respectful of the artworks and the clients and the level of satisfaction and pride the clients felt was evident.

Despite the thorough preparations, the clients sometimes experienced reserved or critical reactions from their friends and even teachers and parents who did not always respond in a supportive and flattering way. There were comments such as: "It's a shame you don't invest that much in your studies" or "It's very nice, but what about your schoolwork." This was an opportunity for a conversation or a comment in the "here and now." I used a variety of responses depending on the situation and upon my professional experience and acquaintance with the clients, their parents and the staff. I often chose to reflect the following message to parents and teachers: "I see that you've noticed how much strength and curiosity he/she has, and you are surprised that there are occasional difficulties in completing homework tasks and class activities." Alternatively I used modeling/reframing. For example: "Today we are happy and excited about their triumphs and achievements. You can see Adam's creativity and strength and maybe we need to think together how we can help Adam feel curious, enthusiastic and interested in academic achievements as well." At other times I chose to relate to things that emerged in our personal art therapy sessions after the exhibition and in the art therapy room. For example, I asked how the student felt about the reaction of a particular friend, teacher or parent and I related to their reaction in the different situations. I also asked: "Is the feeling familiar, how do you usually respond, is it possible to respond in other ways?"

Generally, it was possible to communicate how the students felt to their parents, teachers and friends. Thoughts on more personalized and empowering responses were discussed and we also talked about this issue in broader terms related to their everyday lives. Throughout the process, I tried not to ignore the sense of pride and achievement or the criticism and judgment by the client and the participants in the exhibition. I use these events to explore experiences on the emotional level and to address my clients' coping methods in the past and the present. I capitalized on the educational and therapeutic potential in all the interpersonal interactions that took place at the school and in the art therapy room. This aspect of the exhibition highlights the need to develop a common (unified) language between arts therapists and the educational staff and to devote time to parental guidance during the therapeutic process. Collaboration between the various parties enhances prospects for growth and emotional development, particularly when it comes to primary school students whose return to a healthy developmental path is crucially dependent upon the responses of the family and education systems. The parents and the educational staff serve as agents for change. The focus and reinforcement of positive behaviors and perceptions while reducing negative factors in the system support and facilitate ways to access students' strengths and mobilize them to achieve their therapeutic goals. The functioning of the student depends on both personal and systemic factors.

At the exhibition on recycling, I created a workspace where I placed a large magnetic board alongside a basket of objects which were attached to magnets. The students experimented with creating pictures from the objects, which became an experiential activity for the audience and allowed them to experiment and touch the work materials presented in the exhibition.

As part of the photography exhibit I put a collection of photographs on a table in the exhibit room. Students could choose a photograph at the end of the exhibition and say why they selected it and how they personally related to it. This experience allowed the teacher to briefly view the emotional sharing experience associated with the therapeutic world. It also enabled the teacher and I to discuss other ways to summarize the process in the classroom and gave an opportunity to start discussions about classroom students. The teachers often provided me with important information and insights about clients that enabled me to maintain and continue my work with them. The principal, counselor, school psychologist, teachers, school maintenance man and security guard were all invited to the exhibition and their presence at the exhibition was important to my clients.

The parents' different ways of reacting to the exhibition were particularly interesting. The respectful, thorough and serious way in which the artworks were presented elicited sensitive, complimentary and supportive responses from the parents. The students were pleased to see their parents' appreciation and admiration, and the festive atmosphere at the end of the year provided me with another opportunity to see the progress that every one of my clients and their parents had made. They had learned to respond from a less critical and a more sensitive, distinct place. During the concluding conversations with parents at the end of the school year, I usually describe the process, achievements, difficulties and future goals, whereas here the students were given a unique opportunity to experience their parents' gaze that Winnicott (1971) described and praised. Winnicott (1971) believed that there is no observed object and there is no creation without the observer. The perception of the observer generates the object. He claimed that the baby reflected in his/her mother's eyes sees him/herself reflected in the mother's loving and admiring gaze. Winnicott described the maternal gaze and its role in establishing the infant's existence; whoever sees the infant, enables the infant to grow. During the parental guidance process, I realized that for some parents, the exhibition, which expressed their children's creativity and skill, allowed them to feel that they were being perceived in a different context than when they came to school for a conference with the teachers or myself, in a situation where we were all focused solely on their children's achievements.

Mango (2001) discussed the involvement of families in a client exhibition in the US as part of Mental Illness Awareness Week. The clients stated that their relatives' attitudes towards them changed for the better after they visited the exhibition. They described how members of their families were able to see their praiseworthy abilities. Many family members talked about their feelings of pride and joy. The art therapist reported that family members who were involved in the therapeutic process gained in various ways from participating in the exhibition and their involvement in the clients' lives took on further dimensions. In addition, the clients whose family members did not attend the exhibition still benefitted from the emotional support and a sense of family from the visitors and staff who attended the exhibition. The reactions of other clients who participated in the exhibition made them feel pleased and proud. Thus, the emotional support that they received from members of their community contributed and promoted a broader perspective with regard to individuals coping with mental illnesses and challenged some of the stereotypes related to members of the community.

These exhibits also led to a change in some of the parents and their parenting from a sense of helplessness, where at times they had withdrawn from their responsibilities and passed them on to the professionals. Instead, during the exhibit, the educational staff and I looked at them with admiration. These moments were documented in photographs taken during the exhibit where family members stood together and hugged each other next to the artworks and showed their sense of pride, pleasure and admiration.

Step Five – the Process Summary – dismantling and Reassembling a Personal Narrative

The summary of the process, the dismantling of the exhibition and the rearrangement of the room are often accompanied by feelings of emotional density that typically characterize the goodbyes at the end of every school year. The story of Avi, a sixth-grade student, is a good example. During his early childhood, his father was absent for a long period of time, but in recent years has returned to fulfill his role as a father figure. Avi formed a meaningful relationship with his teacher and progressed substantially both socially and educationally. However, at home he occasionally behaved aggressively towards his mother and refused to obey authority and accept boundaries, forcing his father to come to their home to "help" Avi's mother deal with the complex situation. Avi wanted his parents to be together again and used his obstinate behavior to "force" his divorced parents to be in continuous dialogue and work collaboratively. Additionally, Avi's glorification of his father emerged in therapy. Avi never mentioned his father's absence or any difficulties in their relationship. In the exhibit, he presented a battleship carrying a tank (see Figure 10.1). In a story that he wrote about the ship, he talked about a commander who abandoned his soldiers. Throughout the therapeutic process, Avi could not understand or make the connection between the powerful defenses that appeared in the form of the battleship and soldiers and the story of disappointment in the "commander who abandoned his crew."

While we were arranging the room after the exhibition was dismantled, I spoke to Avi and asked him: "How do you feel at the end of the exhibition?"

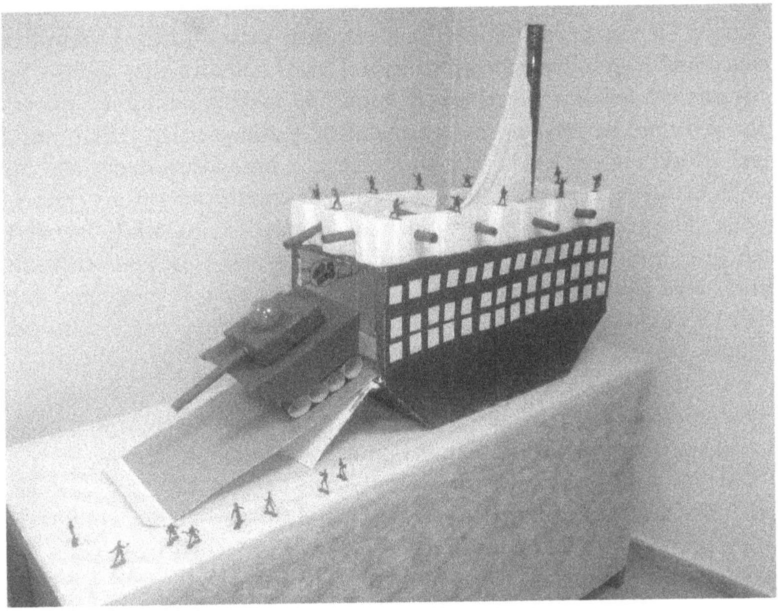

Figure 10.1 The Trojan Ship.

Avi: "It was fun. Mother came to see the exhibition and father didn't."

Me: "What did you think, and feel?"

Avi: "Father always makes promises and never keeps them. At home he also promises to come pick me up after work and doesn't come. He often says that he will stop getting angry, but he never does."

I was very surprised by Avi's honesty and openness. This was a month before the termination of his therapeutic process. He felt brave enough to talk for the first time about his disappointment from his father. I reflected this to him: "You seem disappointed and you feel that this is not the first time he has broken his promise."

Avi: "Yes, this is true" (with a sad expression).

Me: "It seems that it is harder to be angry at Father, with Mommy it is easier."

Avi smiled.

At the end of the process, we talked about his disappointment and his aggression directed at his mother. Together we decided that the artwork that he displayed in the exhibition and planned to take to his father's house would remain in the art therapy room and that I would keep it for him. I suggested that we take photographs of his artwork from different angles for him to have as a memento. The realization that his father was unable to keep his artwork at home was significant. Avi's prior idealization of his father stopped aiding him and led him to enact more effective defense mechanisms.

Another example is Daniel, who had been in art therapy from third to sixth grade. He was a curious, intelligent student with a learning disability and considerable graphomotor difficulties. Daniel had difficulty socializing and his anxiety levels were relatively high. He made significant progress and showed marked improvement academically and socially. There was a decrease in his anxiety levels, and an increase in his independence and his ability to organize, plan and execute his artwork with the various creative materials. The conversation took place in a group setting while we were dismantling the exhibition. Daniel inquired several times whether the students were frightened and afraid of the snakes that he presented and whether he was able to trick the viewers into thinking they were real snakes (see Figure 10.2).

Me: "Yes, mostly the little kids kept asking if the snakes were real."

Daniel smiles with an expression of satisfaction.

Me: "Did you want to scare the children?"

Daniel: "Yes, snakes remind people of death and things like that. I like seeing scary things and I have stories that I wrote when I was younger, scary stories. Some of them are about snakes and the grim reaper, and they usually had a happy ending. For some reason I am drawn to this

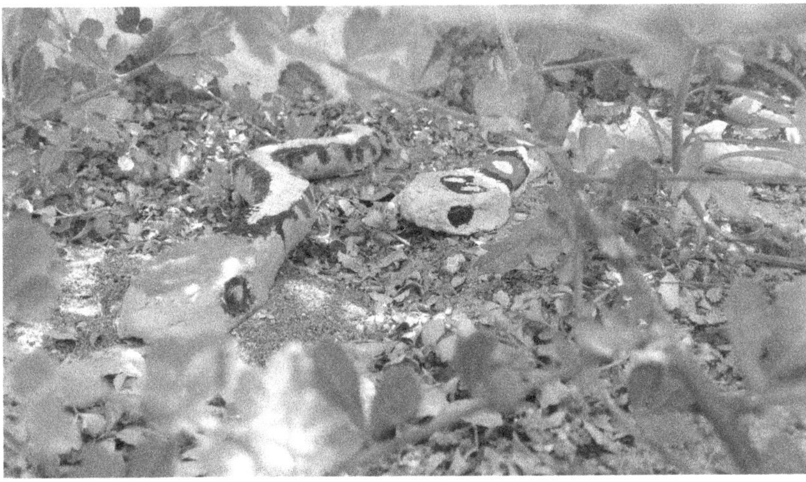

Figure 10.2 Fears.

subject. When I was small, I was a bit of a scaredy-cat and now I don't really feel the fear. I remember that I had panic attacks and that I got out of bed and I was scared. But I understood that it was nonsense from my imagination."

Simon: (his friend from the group): "I am still afraid of some things....That something will happen to my parents, that someone will hurt me, that I'll get stuck in an elevator."

Daniel: "And you are constantly playing scary games on the computer, maybe you should stop."

Simon: "Yes, I think that I should stop."

I noticed that the process of dismantling the exhibition and the concluding remarks made it possible to connect to a deeper internal layer. The process allowed for the formation of emotional connections which for Simon had been more elusive. "The function of the inner witness" (Amir, 2013) allows an individual to tell his/her own story and personal narrative that includes a historical sequence. It is also about self-observation and the ability to validate one's subjective experience. As part of the exhibition, the experience is validated not only by me, the students' art therapist, but also by the educational staff and peer group.

When the dismantling was over, we sat together in a group and used emotion cards with photographs. I asked the group to describe the work process (preparation, exhibition and end of process). Or, a fourth grader, shared his personal experience with us. He expressed the conflict that he felt very deeply; on the one hand, he spoke of the need to be seen and the desire to share his experience of accomplishment with his friends and educational staff (as a student who often struggles with emotional regulation and discipline problems) but on the other, he described his fear and shame. Or described it this way in response to figures taken from POINTS OF YOU (see Figures 10.3–10.5: **Photos from Punctum Game by Points of You®**)

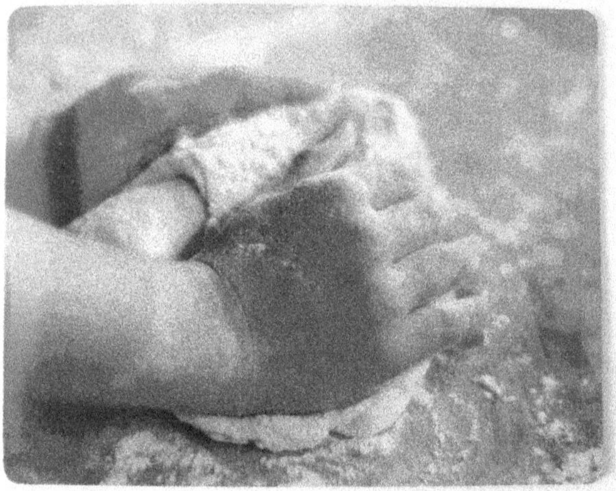

Figure 10.3 "We Worked Hard."

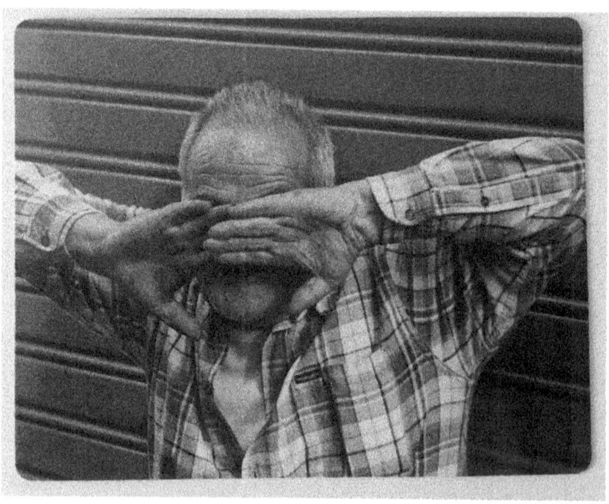

Figure 10.4 "I Was Ashamed."

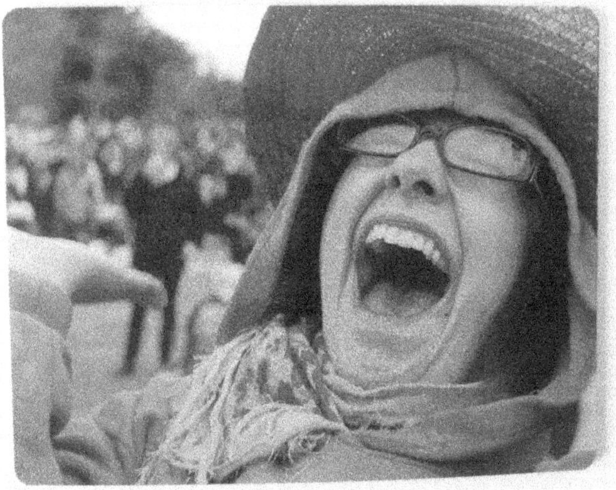

Figure 10.5 "And People Said Wow."

His pleasure and satisfaction with the entire process was palpable. His emotions clearly and distinctly expressed the start of his internalization of the gap that he experienced between his vastly different way of functioning in the art therapy room and in the classroom. I hope that Or continues to learn to regulate his emotions and that his creative strengths and self-awareness will assist him in the process of growth and change.

Summary and Conclusions

From my personal standpoint, the school should be used as a therapeutic, educational and social setting that provides each client with the opportunity to develop emotionally in all its spaces. Every interpersonal interaction that occurs within the school space has both educational and therapeutic potential. This underscores the need to craft a unified language that engages the cooperation of all role holders. In a study by Snir and colleagues (2018), they mention that art therapists are often perceived by the educational staff as misunderstood and uninvolved, and the art therapists struggle to feel a sense of belonging with the school framework. As shown here, the decision to hold the exhibition in the school space and invite all the staff members to be active viewers allowed me to become more integrated into the system, feel that I belonged to the framework and enable the educational team to better understand me.

With the help of formal and informal staff interactions, we were able to contain and deal with the complexities of the splitting mechanism. Winnicott (1984) states that teachers who work with anti-social children are in practice functioning as group mental health therapists who add a touch of teaching to their work. I believe this statement is valid and extremely important to the education system. Our role as arts therapists is to contribute to the educational team not only via our empathic abilities but also through our experience and professional knowledge. We need to participate and, when necessary, guide and advise staff how to respond and cope with the challenges and experiences that students face.

This collaboration allows the educational and therapeutic team to experience a sense of ability. This in turn is likely to lead to an increase in their ability to contain and enable more effective coping with the many challenges that students face. Since many of my clients significantly lack the representations of "others" and an experience of the "self" when participating in meaningful interpersonal relationships, it is important for these clients to have many "others" so that all clients in their own way can have many types of experiences and events from which to find the individuals who will accept and enable them to learn and change negative internal models and thereby take responsibility for their role in society.

The different exhibitions expressed the creative thinking of the entire system. This conceptualization always involved calculated risks, feeding the imagination and exploring new ideas. Robinson (2011) noted that a creative organization allows for risk taking and serves as a place that permits its employees to develop their own insights, encourages inquiry, and values those who are dynamic, surprising and test the boundaries. I believe it is possible to expand, adapt and deepen the school space to contain the "intermediate space" within it. The exhibition and other initiatives can serve as a bridge and milestone for the educational team, as well as an invitation to become "significant" partners in a space where, on the one hand, there is an understanding of the importance of reality, which is usually expressed by teachers, and on the other, a locus of encounter between inner and outer reality, where fantasy and reality are intermingled by the arts therapist. This mental space, which lies halfway between an objective reality and a subjective experience, is the basis for both creativity and the ability to expand the concrete everyday experience.

I believe that meaningful education requires flexibility and, in particular, an invitation to experiment, explore and learn who we are and not only study different subjects. The therapeutic process is saturated with conflicting needs: stability versus personality growth, maintaining privacy and individuality in the face of the need to share with others and continuity of self-experience in the face of change. I am aware of the widespread professional debate about exposing artworks from the art therapy room in the public space. The purpose of this chapter was to reinforce the benefits of taking a flexible view of clients' needs and to adapt the norms associated with the potential space. The art therapists' partnerships and initiatives aimed at the client's progress will improve their chances of expanding their support circles and recruiting the educational staff for assistance. Exhibitions are another way to connect and create a bridge between art therapists and the educational staff, as well as respond to the emotional needs of the clients.

References

Amir, D. (2013). *Cleft tongue*. Jerusalem: Magnes (in Hebrew).

Chambala, M.A. (2008) Anxiety and art therapy: treatment in the public eye. *Art Therapy: Journal of the American Art Therapy Association*, *25*(4), 187–189.

Govrin, A. (2013). *Conservative and radical perspectives on psychoanalytic knowledge: The fascinated and the disenchanted*. New York: Routledge.

Johnson, E. R. (2013). Patient art exhibitions in health care settings. In C. A. Malchiodi (Ed.*), Art therapy and health care* (pp. 333–346). New York: The Guilford Press.

Leenstra, S., Goldstraw, S., & Rumbold, B. (2014). Art as evidence: Ethical considerations when using client artworks in exhibitions. *Journal of Applied Arts & Health*, *5*(2), 227–234.

Mango, C. (2001). Art on my mind. *Art Therapy*, *18*(4), 216–219.

Osterville, Z. (1995). *Open solutions: The psychological treatment of children*. Tel Aviv: Schocken Publishing House (in Hebrew).

Rand, V. (2011) Ethics on exhibit. *Art Therapy: Journal of the American Art Therapy Association*, *28*(4) ,152–158.

Robinson, K. (2011). *Out of our minds*. Tantor Media, Incorporated.

Snir, S., Regev, D., Keinan, V., Abd El Kader-Shahada, H., Salamey, A., Mekel, D., … Alkara, M. (2018). Art therapy in the Israeli education system–a qualitative meta-analysis. *International Journal of Art Therapy*, *23*(4), 169–179.

Weinfeld Yehudian, O. (2013). Unique characteristics of therapeutic work in an open space – the arts therapies in a hospital for pediatric hemodialysis. *Academic Journal of Creative Arts Therapies*, *3*, 273–285 (in Hebrew).

Winnicott, D. (1971). *Playing and reality*. New York: Basic Books.

Winnicott, D. W. (1984). *Deprivation and delinquency*. New York: Tavistock.

11 CoAT

A Community-based Therapeutic Approach in Educational Environments

Efrat Roginsky, Tamar Sade-Dor, Osnat Dvir, Yael Halahmi and Sandra Goldman

Introduction

Arts therapists in the Israeli education system adhere to a predefined policy of inclusion (Snir et al, 2018). Students diagnosed with diverse learning and health conditions are entitled to educational, functional, behavioral, emotional and social services to ensure their inclusion in school. The latter are mainly accommodated by arts therapists, through arts psychotherapy[1] (Snir et al, 2018) which takes place individually, in pairs or small groups in designated rooms at school. Arts psychotherapy has a specific language, ethics and guidelines, which differ from the school's educational discourse in many ways. At times, arts therapists face misunderstanding and mistrust as a result of these differences (Belity, Regev, & Snir, 2016).

Many contemporary arts therapies derive from the medical, educational and rehabilitation fields. For a few decades the emphasis was on psychodynamic theories. More recently, additional approaches have evolved within the arts therapies in response to the broad range of users[2], settings, policies and financing systems (see Bolger, Skewes-McFerran, & Stige, 2018). This variety of perspectives does not necessarily contradict but rather complements and demonstrates the many possible benefits of the arts for individuals' well-being (see McFarren, Thompson, & Bolger, 2015). Community Arts Therapies (CoAT[3]) (Animbom-Ngong, 2017; Ansdell, 2002; Ottemiller-Drusedum & Awais, 2016) are an example of one contemporary approach. The purpose of this chapter is to describe CoAT in terms of their origins, theoretical foundations and key principles. Schools are seen as micro-communities, the idea of school-CoAT is presented and CoAT's potential with respect to inclusion in education is discussed.

CoAT are not prevalent in Israeli schools; the arts-therapist authors of this chapter were not informed by this approach, but came to espouse it intuitively as a way to accommodate their users' needs, or in response to various professional challenges. Four case studies are presented; each is followed by insights and thoughts on school-CoAT. Visual art therapists as well as a music therapist primarily collaborated on this chapter. This influenced our choices of the literature and case studies; however, we suggest that CoAT, due to their meta-theoretical perspective, is not necessarily limited to visual arts or music. The conclusion touches on the potential and challenges of CoAT, as reflected through the case studies and the therapists' experiences.

Theoretical Background

Community Arts Therapies

Over the last few decades, the arts therapies professions have evolved rapidly. Initially, many of these professions were based on the medical model and psychotherapeutic theories (Malchiodi, 2005). Today, arts therapists use a broader range of approaches, including the social model of disability (Oliver, 2013), as well as concepts related to empowerment, well-being and health (Baines, Pereira, Hatch, & Edwards, 2019; Stige, Ansdell, Elefant, & Pavlicevic, 2010). Community-oriented arts therapies (CoAT) derive from these approaches (Huss, Kaufman, Avgar, & Shuker, 2016; Stige, Ansdell, Elefant, & Pavlicevic, 2010) and focus on the potential of service-users rather than their challenges (Aigen, 2014). At-risk groups or refugees are reported to have benefitted from this therapeutic approach (Stige Stige, Ansdell, Elefant, & Pavlicevic, 2010).

Like any arts therapies approach, CoAT require a comprehensive setting, ethical guidelines, careful management and professional supervision. Here, however, these parameters can vary considerably as a function of each community of users and in particular their culture, environment, challenges, potentials and the goals of therapy (Aigen, 2014; Pavlicevic, 2004). The artistic media are always at the core of CoAT (Aigen, 2014); Ansdell (2002) even suggested calling community music therapists "therapeutic musicians in residence" (para. 2) to highlight their specific professional identity, as well as the powerful role of the arts. The nature of therapeutic relations in CoAT can vary in definition and nature depending on the culture and the needs of the therapy-users and can include co-artists or musicians, coaches, stage directors, producers and others (Aigen, 2014). In all cases, mutuality is encouraged. CoAT do not focus exclusively on the improvement of individual users, but rather views their development as embedded within a social network and context such that the development of the whole community can enhance the inclusion and health of its members (Davies, Richards, & Barnwick, 2015). Hence, these features are nurtured in CoAT, and artistic processes and products are sometimes introduced to even broader, external social circles such as the class, family and neighborhood (Huss et al., 2016; Stige et al., 2010).

Elefant (2016) described community music therapy with a choir of physically challenged members; the shared experience and ongoing dialogue turned this choir into a small, supportive community, where each member had his or her own identity and expression. Huss et al. (2016)

described the influences of community visual art therapy on victims of war and disaster areas and noted that therapy afforded the expression of their traumatic experiences as well as mutual support. In later stages, there was a sense of communal regeneration. Elefant (2016) promoted the inclusion of special-education students in their hometown communities through music sessions with another group of school children.[4] Mutual curiosity and cooperation developed, as well as parental support for the children's continuing contacts.

These brief examples show that CoAT can contribute not only to traumatized individuals or those marginalized by society but also be effective in more normative settings such as schools, as is exemplified in the case studies below (Elefant, 2016; McFerran & Rickson, 2014). CoAT are examined in this article not as a substitute, but rather as a complementary approach in schools, alongside other arts psychotherapies.

School – Community

A community (from Latin: commun) describes a social group with some definitions or characteristics in common, varying across the span of history, and different fields of knowledge (Community, 2019). Zachary (2012) argued that communities are characterized by collaborative interaction, a distinct geographic territory, shared values, beliefs or behaviors. Turner (1969) used the Latin term "Communitas" (p. 360) to distinguish any ordinary gathering of people from a meaningful, even sacred sense of being together. In the context of Community Music Therapy (CoMT), Ansdell (2004) reported how the ongoing creation and performance of music (Musicking) gave rise to a sense of communitas (or, "communication-community") (pp. 44–47). In CoAT, we suggest that meaningful community-communication through artistic media is the main source of communitas.

Many schools consider that part of their mission is to serve their surrounding communities, and that families share their everyday, mutual values and cultures. Harpaz (2014) termed these schools "communities of thinking" to denote the ongoing student-teacher dialogue. Friedman (1990) suggested that schools should be open to various forms of discourse from the community and the authorities. Our perspective is similar, and hence, in this chapter, we consider schools as communal facilities.

Traditional Arts Therapies in Israeli Schools

Around the globe, inclusion in education secures the right of students with diverse conditions to care and support within their local education systems. Specialized educational as well as therapeutic staff members are hired to respond to this goal (Inclusive education, 2019). However, inclusion may generate challenges since different students may require special approaches and modes of communication that are not always within the realm of possibility of the school staff, students or parents (Talmor, Reiter, & Feigin, 2004). The diversity of the student can also lead to exclusion and loneliness. Arts therapists can engage schools in developing more awareness and tools to overcome exclusion, but psychological approaches to therapy also face a number of obstacles within school environments in particular as regards the language of therapy and the ethical commitment related to the therapeutic alliance (Snir et al., 2018), the emotional shift involved in the transition from class to therapy room, the disruption of therapy by school programs and vacations and insufficient parental involvement. Psychotherapy by nature is aimed at specific users, which may identify them at school as impaired. In contrast, a community-based approach supports inclusion as a result of its ecological framework, culture-conscious language and the use of school's everyday environment. CoAT do not designate any children as impaired and harness their potential for the greater good. To illustrate, below we present several pioneering case studies from the work of four school art therapists.

Description of the Working Model and Clinical Examples

The cases described here were not deliberately conceived as CoAT but were more an experimental outcome of the work the art therapists engaged in them. Each case is presented briefly, followed by our thoughts regarding its community characteristics and its influence on the school environment.

Yael Halahmi – inclusion through an Art Therapy Group

This case study describes a therapy group, initially no different from many others, that was gradually shaped to become more community-aware. The therapy process is described, and its CoAT characteristics are highlighted.

The group. The setting was a small second grade at a large local school that only had one special education class. The students had a range of developmental, behavioral and emotional challenges and came from different socioeconomic backgrounds. Although efforts had been devoted to therapy, limited attention had been paid to the children's inclusion in the school community. The parents of these students initially asked the staff to devote more time to their children's inclusion and participation in the school's social life. The homeroom teacher was enthusiastic but felt she needed to prepare the students by reinforcing their social skills and confidence.

It was decided to create a social-skill group that I, the visual art therapist, would co-lead with the school counselor. The initial plan was to integrate the special education students with a few additional second graders. We were both in charge of organizing the group; we held a regular weekly consultation, as well as scheduled meetings with the teacher. Four students and two students from another class were chosen, all of whom were challenged behaviorally. Co-direction of this complex group felt safer, and the regular meetings with the teacher broadened our perspective on the process. Working so closely together enhanced our professional skills and led to deeper collegial relations.

The setting. We met 45 minutes weekly, in the school's art therapy room, for a total of 25 sessions overall. The objectives were to cultivate the children's social skills, enterprise and leadership, provide regulation training, nurture their self-confidence and a sense of belonging. We hoped that the group activity and our mediation would give the special education students an opportunity to relate to the other second graders safely. The therapy sessions were highly structured with respect to the children's challenges. They began with a physical warm-up, and social activities in a circle or in pairs demanding attention and attunement. Then, we had artistic creation, a verbal discussion, art presentations and clean up at the end. There was also a regular closing ceremony.

The therapeutic process. During the first session, the participants were introduced to each other and the therapy room, and together we agreed on a code of behavior. For the subsequent sessions, the children created sock hand-puppets, and they suggested building a Punch and Judy theater. This project required a great deal of cooperation, and genuine friendships emerged within our group. When the puppet theater was ready, personal stories, free-play and deeper relations evolved. At times, disputes and conflicts occurred, but through the co-guidance, the artistic media, as well as our code of behavior, these could be resolved without aggressiveness.

Later, we created group-mandalas. The shared work generated issues of belonging and inclusion versus the fear of exclusion, and the children's wish for separate identities. Our final sessions were dedicated to the upcoming separation; we examined the artistic creations, held a group exhibition and created an album for each child through which the children could process their group experiences.

The outcome. As a preparatory step for broader inclusion of the special education class at school, the children's social skills were addressed. The art therapy group indeed afforded an intimate, safe atmosphere where acquaintance was made with the other second graders, and deeper relations immerged. The children's separate identities were nurtured, as was their ability to participate through play, motion, creation and words. The leaders' mediation allowed the students to perceive and accept each other. Their social flexibility and mutual play improved, as well as the verbal, age-appropriate expression of their emotions. In the schoolyard, the confidence and intimacy between our group of participants were evident; at school recesses they would play spontaneously, and even join other students with growing enthusiasm.

The co-guidance of the group afforded us to contain its challenging participants and provide them with a model for teamwork. The class-staff also considered this group setting as an opportunity to share our multiprofessional experience, and establish deep, supportive team relations.

Analysis in terms of CoAT. This experience adhered to the community therapeutic approach in a number of ways, as described below.

Nonhierarchical collaboration. The cooperative work of parents, teachers, assistive and therapeutic staff regarding the students' inclusion was unusual at this school. It arose out of teamwork, and not from the efforts of a single therapist alone.

Attending to the need to belong. The basic human need to participate and interact (Foulks, 1974) was one of the prime motivators for the creation of this group. The parents, as primary partners, identified the class as segregating, separating and disruptive of their children's social development; their opinion was taken seriously by the staff. This wish to break through the barriers of exclusion was also echoed in the staff's improved teamwork and deepening relations.

Focusing on the user's potential. This was the first time these students were perceived through their abilities, not challenges. Their rapid social development during this year validated this approach. Nurturing the children's ability to dialogue and play in an age-appropriate manner facilitated their greater engagement at recess time.

Art-centered process. The group experiences were based on collaborative artistic work. The art encouraged interpersonal exploration, as well as the expression of thoughts and ideas even before they were mentalized or discussed within the group. The creative process and products allowed the children to experience deep involvement, enthusiasm and play. It was a source of mutual pride and living proof of the students' abilities.

Tamar Sade-Dor – "Our Song" Group

The following case study describes the transition from a personalized form of therapy to a classroom setting that included the students and some staff members. Multidisciplinary cooperation is highlighted and discussed. The arts were once again the core of therapy and served to bridge between the students and participating staff members.

The background. I was involved with the ninth and final grade of junior high school for this special education class. I had known some of the students through previous individual therapy, in pairs, or small groups in the therapy room. Towards graduation, I felt the urge to do something new to demarcate the special spirit of this year. After discussing some ideas at a staff meeting, it was decided to form a whole-class therapy group, led by the homeroom teacher, the counselor and me. Our assigned goal was to deal with the class as a whole during its last year at school by encouraging greater awareness and active discussions. The staff was curious about therapy work and would often say they would like to be a fly on my wall in the art therapy room. They now had the opportunity to experience the therapeutic language and the students' worlds more closely. This mutual work also reduced my own isolation within this large educational facility.

The setting and therapeutic process. We introduced the class to our idea of designing an artistic graduation project to be presented at school. This idea was soon postponed and replaced with a slower start where the students and staff would re-introduce themselves to each other by listening to their favorite songs. We called the group "our song" to reflect this idea. Our aim was to empower each student, encourage responsibility, reinforce team spirit and practice age-appropriate social skills, all of which are suitable goals for the graduation year.

Weekly, 45-minute sessions were held around a large U-shaped table in class. On the table, we put felt-tipped pens, Artline, oil pastels and colored pencils of several sizes. Each time, a different student or staff member would share her or his favorite song. We listened together, and then shared our experiences and thoughts. After a discussion, we would all draw our experiences from the music on a plain A4 piece of paper. The artwork was shared, with or without commentary, and a second discussion was generated. At the end of each session, the next presenter of a song was chosen. Towards the end of the year and the end of our process, each participant chose a single artwork, and we discussed these choices. These works were used to form a shared collage constituting a larger collaborative piece of art. Together we added, changed and combined each other's artworks. At the end we introduced modeling clay. By smearing, all the separate parts of the work were highlighted, covered and connected, and new elements were formed.

The co-leading. Initially, the leaders' tasks were quite distinct. I managed the group, whereas the teacher and counselor were in charge of the behavior and the rules. Together, we found a way to communicate, associate and sum up each session. The teacher frequently suggested more practical ideas: "Why did you do so, and not the other way?" "Is anything missing in your drawing?" The counselor encouraged the students' verbalization: "Can you say a bit more?" "Was there anything else that you could say about it?" I would try to calm the students' fears of exposure, but still encourage authentic behavior and expression: "It's all right," I would say, "Don't force yourself to talk today, your art speaks better than words." As the group process continued, our voices and roles were more integrated. As time passed, we felt the lack of regular staff meetings since we had no place to process our reflections, thoughts or future plans.

The class process. Our lesson and ideas seemed strange to the students at first, but after some time they adjusted. The work in words, music and visual art afforded a multifaceted encounter, and each student participated in her or his own way. Most of them engaged in music and visual art. The structured setting was safe and intimate. They created with a growing depth of emotions and themes; feelings and ideas were shared, and the students took on more leadership within this group. As challenging matters emerged, we would make sure that everyone felt safe. We paid separate attention when issues were more private and complex. By the end of this year, a broad range of personal and group processes could be seen from the work.

Towards the end of this year, the work slowed down. The sessions were freer and more intuitive, and we did not seem to have achieved the initial goal of sharing the artistic outcome with others. The collective artwork was not completed given school vacations, activities and the lack of regular staff meetings. Finally, it was decided to give each group member a photograph of the collaborative artwork. The last staff meeting on the group enabled us to process its significance and influence on everyday activities in the class. We thought that similar projects would require a long-term plan that was better adapted to the school setting and school calendar and would have more regular staff meetings. We discussed the advantages of visual art, music and words in this process. Currently additional groups are being planned for similar and even younger students, with an improved organization and setting.

Analysis in terms of CoAT: The following characteristics of the "our-song" group coincided with the community therapeutic approach.

Professional collaboration. This is an example of a broader multiprofessional collaboration than the first case study (art therapist and counselor). The integrated, direct work with the students on the part of three staff members and therapists reinforced our understanding, involvement and intervention in this class. Empowerment was provided not only to the students but also to us, the staff members, and enabled mutual development and learning.

Whole class treatment. Traditional psychotherapy tends to question the benefits of classroom treatment. Our experience showed that a secure and intimate space was established successfully. Even though some students were previously in the therapist's care, the classwork seemed efficient and was highly appreciated. The class setting and friends made may have even improved the students' ability to engage with others.

Preplanned process and product. CoAT are arts-centered, and sometimes product-centered. Often, a project or product is designed with a preplanned schedule, which in our case was the structured artwork, and the proposed presentation of the collective work by the end of this year. These elements were meant to provide a safe space for processing the upcoming separation upon graduation, but also to reconnect to the students' wider context of families and the school from which they would part through the presentation. Indeed, this structure afforded a rich discussion, a mentalization of ideas and mutual processing. Towards the end of this year, we reconsidered the broader-scale presentation. We had a few clinical and practical discussions regarding this transition, but in the end, we decided not to do the presentation. Flexibility was allowed to correspond to the group's feelings regarding their privacy, their work pace and the relations with their broader community at this time. Despite being art and product-centered, CoAT are closely attuned to their users' context and needs; this may be what distinguishes community arts therapies from community-arts[5].

The staff participation in art. The therapist's deliberate participation in the artwork is more common in CoAT than it is in psychotherapy (Ansdell, 2002). In this class, we believed that more equal relations could improve the students' trust and engagement. In fact, closeness and intimacy seemed to encourage the group in that our visual ideas were sometimes echoed in the students' art, and the group would see and discuss these issues of similarity and differences as part of their ongoing developmental process.

Sandra Goldman – including Drop-out Students in an Art Therapy Group

This case study deals with a small art therapy group that was held in the school yard and was intended to contribute to the whole community and not only a few specific users. The school's ecology was essential to our work and included the students, the staff, the school culture and the environment.

The background. For a few years I worked as a visual art therapist at a small elementary school. Many children came from economically deprived families, and others from Ethiopian immigrant families that were still dealing with issues of their social identity and social status. In this school, many children simply left in the middle of class and tended to wander around the school yard. This was so pervasive and disturbing that yard supervisors were hired to engage with the children to prevent violence and vandalism.

At that time, I only worked with children entitled to art therapy. Many other children at school were not provided therapy because of their parents' lack of understanding of the eligibility process, their level of language proficiency as non-native speakers of Hebrew or lack of money to pay for professional diagnoses. Given the number of students not in class and as a witness to its deleterious influences on the community and environment, I felt I should make therapy more accessible for these children as well. Art therapy as I see it does not necessarily require a private space; rather, creative processes can also occur in the open. I thought that working in the yard might encourage these children to participate as well. I planned to construct a core group of therapy-entitled children, with greater behavioral and dialoguing abilities. This group would go from the therapy room out to the school yard frequently and be engaged in social-ecological activism. This group's work, I thought, could encourage some of the children dropping out of class to take part in our creative work.

The setting. Six children of different ages and backgrounds participated in the core group; all of them were facing social challenges and had low self-esteem. I was in charge and was helped by an 18-year-old girl doing her mandatory stint in the army through public service. We had 90 weekly minutes throughout the school year. This group's main goal was to empower its participants, and to contribute to the school environment and community. The participants were engaged in project-planning, problem-solving and collaborative work, for the good of their whole community.

Most of these children had been working with me more traditionally; when I told them about my new ideas for the group, they asked to discuss it more fully. One especially vulnerable child could not sustain this loss of intimacy or the exposure of our work in the schoolyard and he was moved to a more conservative therapy group. The other participants in the core group felt they could cope with the changes. Just as in this first session, it was essential for me that the students' voices be heard, and their plans translated into acts and products. Going out into the broader school setting together, as a group, provided these children with more strength and courage.

The therapeutic process. The initial meetings focused on forming the core group and involved defining rules, boundaries and fostering closer acquaintances. These meetings were held in the art therapy room. During the rest of this year, we spent our time outside in the schoolyard. The therapy room was used chiefly for preparations or processing at the beginning and end of each session. We focused at first on the neglected schoolyard and decided to take time for cleaning, preparing decorative litter bins, but we also had fun such as playing in the mud, creating with paint, clay and other media. We also had social games, just as in the therapy room, but outside. The children and adults passing by were invited to join our work and play. The back and forth motion from therapy room to the yard, and the spontaneous evolution from the core group to a larger one, called for extensive group processes. The changes were discussed in terms of intimacy versus exposure, private versus public. The core group wanted to get closer together, but also they wanted to contribute to helping the other children, the outsiders. The aims of the artistic work were discussed: should they work for their own enjoyment or for the benefit of others? Such topics came up as we worked outside and were processed more intimately at the opening or closing of each session. Nevertheless, the collaborative work and contribution to school were satisfying for all.

Leading the group. I had no co-leaders, mainly because I felt the need to examine this whole new idea on my own at first. The national service volunteer was my assistant during most of this year; she took part in the planning and processing of each session and helped me with the group during our work outside. A young man, who worked in the yard with the drop-out students, would join our sessions, support, create and take part in games. Both partners' warm and accepting presence was of great help to me.

I was truly concerned about experimenting with this new approach that exposed not only the students but also myself and my work to questions and criticism. I was not sure whether the staff or the students would appreciate this new form of therapy, the larger space, the spontaneity and the loss of privacy. I was not sure whether this setting would provide the right mix for expression and growth. This challenging work required a great deal of courage and effort; it was not easy to lead it all by myself. Some of my fears did in fact materialize. The drop-out students joining the group were not always easy to contain in the group. Spontaneous passersby from the staff would sometimes interfere or even scold us; for example, one teacher was not happy to see us playing with mud. Another was worried when we worked outside in the rain. The unfamiliar outcome of the work was also criticized. In these cases, I would always ask myself how to behave, what to say, and I mainly chose not to reply or try to educate and simply keep working. The work itself, I thought, provided a living explanation of what art therapy is, and the art therapy language.

Real-time modeling. When starting the group, I involved senior staff in the planning and setting of the therapy goals. They gave me the autonomy to explore the new therapeutic terrain. During the school year, I preferred to lead the group, and allow our work to be seen and be open to all. This unusual activity in the schoolyard was indeed a powerful call for inquiry and attracted the participation of the children who were out of class as well as the staff. The value of the work to the school was clearly apparent through its visibility and the affordance to participate and experience together.

Anti-model,[6] or the freedom to play. It was enjoyable to leave traditional therapy momentarily and engage in a whole new adventure. No questions or criticism diminished my enthusiasm. The freedom I was granted only energized my therapeutic work. Unlike my isolating work in the therapy room, I enjoyed engaging with my adult assistants; through our work in the yard, we had a chance to experience genuine solidarity and friendship. Even though, or perhaps because our collaboration was largely spontaneous, it was highly attentive and synchronized. We played at and through therapy together. Despite their primary fears, the core group participants reported a sense of empowerment during the mutual work in the yard: here they were, exposed to public view, not the lonely under-achievers they used to be, but a cohesive, contributing group. They cleaned the yard and invited students who were not in class to take part, thus contributing to their community's higher values. The group's games and artwork were seen and appreciated by everyone. The transparent yard work restored these low-achieving students to their school community, with a distinct, more highly appreciated identity. During every session, more students from the yard joined in to engage in the art making and play. Their daily routine at school was very different, since in the past these children would roam around sabotaging equipment, putting themselves at risk or threatening others. When our group worked in the yard, these students did not disturb us; when they approached us, they experienced a warm, sincere welcome from the adults, and later on from the group participants. These newcomers thus experienced inclusion and positive activity.

These community activities were discussed in depth in the core group meetings. The fears, debates and questions took on a new form, and became part of these children's new identity since they felt they were contributing positively to change in their community. This new endeavor was gratifying for me as well; working in the school's public space, not only the therapy room, taught me a great deal and made me feel a deep sense of belonging to this school. Some students still require the intimate therapy room, but I learned that for others, working in their natural environment can enhance treatment, touch on key issues and empower. The school staff also learned more about this different approach to therapy. The principal agreed to supply the resources required for any future group or project. The teachers seemed more inviting and understanding. I ceased to be the alienated person from the therapy room but rather a familiar and accessible figure.

Besides the therapeutic goals we achieved, a sustainable product was left behind in the school yard that constitutes a daily reminder to all my young participants of their abilities and their different potential identities. During the writing of this chapter, a new CoAT group started planning a small sculpture project close to the entrance to the school. In this way, I feel, simply carrying on with the work outside, we can naturally attract more partners and users to create and play, participate and communicate as a broad school community.

In terms of CoAT: The following characteristics correspond to the community therapeutic approach.

Reviving the therapist. This therapist, just as in the previous case study, described a lively process of planning, creation and enjoying the autonomy granted to her in the open school space. She described her satisfaction with spontaneous communication, the chance to develop relationships and the processes occurring during the group's work in the yard. The therapist's role in the artwork gave more depth to her therapeutic perspective and did not sabotage the process in any way.

Flexibility. This therapeutic endeavor was highly dynamic; it shifted repeatedly from the art therapy room to the outside, and from the core group to a larger and spontaneous one. The participants encountered various changes and experiences in the schoolyard. Spontaneity can characterize CoAT, and add a sense of vitality, richness and curiosity. The therapist encouraged this flexibility but was careful to create a safe haven for art therapy through the core group, regular rituals and rules. Importantly, this setting did not suit all the students and required thorough planning and attentiveness.

Transparency. CoAT are sometimes more visible to the surrounding community, especially when inclusion, participation and active influence are part of its main goals. The critique and the questions addressed by observers, the close relations and mutual learning established with the community members involved were essential in this therapeutic perspective. The therapist's ability to explain or demonstrate the treatment, its ideas, aims and actions were critical for this therapy's success.

Empowerment. Supporting the users' abilities, motivations and achievements in their own surrounding is fundamental in this therapeutic paradigm; in this case, the core group children were seen and benefitted from their care of the school environment and their fellow students. They were viewed not as special education students receiving therapy, but as active, contributing community members. The drop-out students had had the chance to experience cooperation, inclusion and respect when they joined the CoAT group. The privacy of therapy room would have not afforded such experiences.

Osnat Dvir – the Eco-Garden Farewell

This therapeutic project was influenced in part by the CoAT approach. Our special-education sixth grade had entered the last year of primary school, and we were looking for ideas for a sustainable farewell project that would present this class respectfully and embrace it as part of the school community. This case study describes the experiences of the students and staff during our CoAT transition from the therapy room to the school's public space.

The background. I had worked with this special education class since their first grade. The class was composed of 15 students, their homeroom teacher, the class assistant and various other staff members. These students came from different towns in the area, and faced various academic, behavioral and social challenges. During the previous years I had worked with these students individually, in pairs or small groups. Towards graduation year, I decided to devote some time to the students' farewell from their class and the school. I felt that five years of art therapy were more than enough for any of these children. It seemed boring and empty, and I wanted the class to engage in new areas of development in a different setting. Our long history together, I thought, was a firm enough base on which to try out new experiences: new spaces, rules, roles and aims in therapy. During all its years at school, this small class had not really participated in the larger school community. I thought that perhaps an art project would enable the students to be more fully present in the public space, contribute to the greater good of school and leave their mark for years to come.

The setting. This was a whole new idea; I needed a great deal of support to promote it at school. I recruited a close colleague; the science teacher who knew these children well and communicated with them easily. This teacher was responsible for the school's ecological garden where every class spent a few hours of work weekly. We decided to situate our project in this garden for the mutual benefit of all the school children. We presented our idea to the homeroom teacher and the school board, where it was approved and funded. The work began.

The whole class took part in planning, choosing an idea and locating the right spot for our project. Throughout this process, they shared their thoughts and emotions regarding possible challenges; each student prepared a draft of what they imagined. The planning stage involved the entire class as well as the teacher, but outside we worked in two groups: each one worked during a different semester.

The science teacher and I co-directed the project. Our cooperation provided a seamless flow from the practical aspects of the work to the more emotional or social issues that followed. Our shared work felt richer than any of my regular art therapy sessions. Each of us had a specific role; this clear definition was useful for the students as well. The class assistant and homeroom teacher supported us in all possible ways, and they took a more active part in our class consultations.

Our primary objectives were as follows:

Develop the students' ability to experience and express themselves in unfamiliar situations or demands.
Encourage them to cope with dynamic social interactions.
Handle frustration and physical challenges.
Encourage initiative and action-taking.
Cultivate their mutual relations.
Reinforce self-esteem and the sense of ability of each student.

The therapeutic process. When we introduced the students to our idea for the project, many of them were enthusiastic, but others found it more problematic; they thought they would miss our closer therapeutic relations. These students were upset and rejected the new idea. The exposure of their work to the whole school, as well as co-creation with such a large group, was hard for them to imagine. During this phase, many ideas and thoughts were shared. The students were concerned about the budget, the weather and their safety. A single provisional idea was chosen by all students in the end that involved building a small meeting place made out of used tires and cement with a bench and a fish pond. Together we went out to the garden and found the right spot for building under a tall tree close to the entrance. In this way anyone entering the eco-garden could see and enjoy it. More drafts were made of the sitting zone and the pond. We looked at all the ideas and discussed every detail. Then construction began. Together we cleared the whole area. We removed rocks, weeds and garbage, and trimmed some branches. Tires were supplied; we filled them with dirt and covered them with concrete. When the bench was ready and dry, we painted and decorated it. The pond was built as well. We documented all the details of our project that was coming to life. Towards the end, we had a concluding conversation in class. The children expressed their feelings and gave some feedback. Some felt successful and proud while others felt that the project had brought them closer to their classmates. Other students shared their ongoing disappointment over the loss of the intimate therapy sessions. As for us, the project leaders, we could see the progress our students had made from an initial lack of belief and low self-esteem to achievement and pride.

We also decided to hold a ceremony to celebrate our new sitting corner in the eco-garden. The students' parents, the school board and staff were invited. Our documentation of the work was presented. Each student received a certificate of honor with a few personal words. The parents were full of pride, and the principal said this project represented the school's flagship of inclusion and integration. We filled the pond with water, and beautiful goldfish were released. Since then, visitors to the school are taken to admire the sitting corner, with much pride.

Main issues in therapy. This group involved labor and dialogue. Some students resisted the dirty, physical work in the garden, and the changing weather conditions; they shared their difficulties as well as other feelings, and then went back to work. The science teacher and I listened; we continuously reflected the children's emotions and tried to find suitable ways for each of them to take part in the project by expressing and creating. There were disagreements over power and control, as well as over tasks and choices, but new friendships also flourished. One student who did not mind hard physical work became the class leader; he took on new responsibilities, distributed tasks and encouraged others who found it harder to cope. Another rejected child cleared the bigger rocks away from the worksite, which required a great deal of physical strength, and this child's newly found ability endowed him with a new identity and role in class. Some students who found the physical labor too challenging were asked to paint and decorate our newly built bench, and two girls prepared a sign with the project name. Everyone in the class found a suitable part to play in our project. It is worth noting that important issues emerged during our work-and-talk process that had never come up during my years of psychodynamic work with the children, such as aggression, leadership, internal struggles, rejection and resistance. The manifestation of these issues was a challenge to us all.

Leading the project. This was an entirely new professional encounter for me that differed considerably from my one-on-one or small group work in the art therapy room. Here I was with the students out in the open, co-leading with a teacher, and coordinated this project closely with numerous staff members and the school board. My continuous presence in the yard also changed my relations with other staff members. My therapeutic work was seen differently in that its goals and outcomes appeared more relevant to the school's daily life. Coming out of their classroom and the therapy room constituted a dramatic change for the special education students as well. They were aided through dialogue that emphasized their service to their whole community. When students and staff passed by, many wanted to lend a hand and the students were glad to receive this help; they suddenly seemed so mature and responsible on their small building site. It was empowering for all of us to present the finished project to the board and parents, which meant a great deal to the whole community.

For me, this mode of working was extremely challenging. I was concerned with ways to overcome the children's anger, disappointment and objections but still allow them a suitable space for development. I found that constantly reflecting and dialoguing can at times be simpler than the vague dynamics of the therapy room. In addition, I was concerned with ways to deal with boundary and behavioral problems in the yard: How should I react? Would I be seen as a teacher, not an art therapist? How would the students cope with my new role? What relations would develop? Because our roles were clearly defined, the students did not seem confused. All of us, I believe, went through development and growth while engaging in this new approach.

In terms of CoAT: The following characteristics corresponded to the community therapeutic approach.

Participation. CoAT can occur in an open, public space. This case study emanated from the school's interest in including and taking pride in its special education class. The process of construction activated two parallel dynamics. The students engaged naturally within their school and community through their weekly work in the yard. The project itself was characterized by creation, initiative and contribution, not weakness. The school's approval, funding and positive feedback made it clear that inclusion was at the top of its agenda.

Summary and Conclusions

These case studies were written by arts therapists who had no previous contact with each other, yet all mention parallel needs and describe intuitions leading to similar solutions. The CoAT approach appeared to motivate lively, integrative work that is extremely pertinent to school environments. Various aspects of community arts therapy were addressed non-theoretically by the therapists, including the human need to belong, the users' health and abilities once given approval and a social context that enables them to flourish, and multiprofessional cooperation on the part of the staff and school boards. The key role of the arts and the pre-defined projects afforded more coherency, security and creativity. Many concerns emerged including the influences of flexible settings, the ongoing transitions from the therapy room to the public areas and the dilemma surrounding the therapist's participation in art. Some goals were achieved with CoAT that would have been more elusive in traditional arts therapies setting; namely, empowerment, participation and inclusion.

All the writers read all the other case studies, as well as the theoretical background to CoAT which they were not familiar. A mutual discussion was initiated in which several key topics emerged.

Psychotherapy or school-CoAT? Due to our minimal experience in CoAT practice and theory, and more extensive involvement in psychotherapeutic approaches, the case studies were deliberately described in simple, universal terms and easy to grasp psychological concepts. We are still in the preliminary stages of examining the advantages and disadvantages of the community therapeutic arts therapies. In any case, we do not consider CoAT to be a substitute for arts therapies at schools, but rather as a complementary approach, to be offered after careful consideration of the environmental and the therapy-users' needs.

Professional identity. CoAT enabled a fundamental shift in professional attitude. The four case studies illustrate the ways in which we successfully overcame our professional isolation at school. Through collaborative work, and intensive, shared consultation with the students and staff, these new identities emerged, as most clearly depicted in Sade-Dor's and in Dvir's cases. Experiences of personal development resulting from cohesive and empathic group work have been discussed extensively in the group analytic literature (for instance, Davies, Richards, & Barwick, 2015, pp. 73–75, 82). As we connected more intensely to a broader social-web, the therapy was not only efficient, but brought about a clear professional shift. Note that we did not experience the community approach as taking over our former identities, but more as accumulating slowly, and added to our existing therapeutic experience.

Increasing the therapist's integration at school. The CoAT work lessened the professional isolation we experienced at school. This isolation was also described in the Snir et al. study (2018). Sade-Dor was able to fulfill her colleagues' wish to witness therapy from within, "like a fly on the wall." Goldman was able to augment her ongoing dialogue with staff members who watched the yard work she led. Halachmi talked about the deepening of relations with her co-leader counselor. In general, we all felt more supported at our schools after the CoAT projects. Halachmi described how the students' group work during recess led to improved integration at school. The use of a community perspective appeared to have improved the dialogue between separate professions, helped clarify the therapeutic work, and involved us more deeply with the schools' staff and mission. This took place without relinquishing our existing professional identities, but rather thorough and mutual experiencing and reflection.

Advancing professional discourse in the arts therapies. All of us felt that CoAT enabled some novel therapeutic possibilities; the artistic media and the close professional collaboration afforded more access to the individual and collective worlds of our therapy-users. The more ecological the work is, including a broader social web of students, staff and parents, the stronger its efficacy. "When our work and dialogue encountered this new terrain, in a large group," Dvir noted, "it allowed me as well as the students to achieve much more than we would in the art therapy room."

CoAT as promoting the user's social inclusion and change. The therapeutic work in public spaces, especially in Dvir's and Goldman's projects, often prompted passers-by to consider the CoAT participants to be privileged. The CoAT students themselves experienced ownership and pride. This response is a strong argument in favor of inclusion at schools in that its application can improve students' motivation to participate in therapy in school.

Challenges, critiques and questions. Breaking through the familiar therapeutic setting and ways of thought also engendered a certain amount of vulnerability. Was this step motivated by our wish to be better acknowledged or more included at school? Were CoAT the best answer to our users' needs? Goldman and Sade-Dor pointed out that it did not suit every child; some sensitive students or topics required a more intimate therapeutic setting. We all agreed that CoAT can be applied as a complementary approach, if found to have more advantages than other forms of arts therapies.

Can CoAT function as an independent therapeutic approach? There is scant literature on community art therapies. Studies have yet to assess the number of therapists using this perspective, and the extent to which they draw on the literature. Ansdell (2002) reported that some music therapists were hesitant to disclose their community interventions; this was also our concern at times. In our opinion, embarrassment or a lack of knowledge can only make CoAT a lightweight, experimentally undeveloped approach. Thus, we strongly recommend continuing to apply, study and write in this field. Currently there is more literature on community-based music therapy; hence, we suggest expanding research and practice to other modalities as well. In this manner, a truly influential body of knowledge can be formed.

Will public school systems apply CoAT regularly? The answer to this question also depends on further experience, research and scholarly work, as well as policies and politics. This short chapter points to the various advantages deriving from school CoAT. Nevertheless, more research is needed on its influences and the resources required to apply them in schools systematically. Other questions that call for further study include: How does it feel, working as a CoAT therapist at school, experimenting, and exposed, coping with a larger number of users, and a complex professional dialogue? When schools themselves discover the benefits of CoAT, will they continue to encourage more traditional forms of arts psychotherapy? Can arts therapists easily adopt multidisciplinary psychotherapeutic and CoAT identities as a function of their users' needs? These issues, as well as the lack of a standard ethical code in community approach, can still limit the regular use of CoAT in schools.

Ansdell (2002) also described community music therapy as an "anti-model"; this idea may trouble any arts therapist wishing to experiment with CoAT in school. Another concern is the lack of professional education and support for CoAT therapists. Sade-Dor noted in conclusion that

> CoAT schoolwork is very exciting and different. When the school is supportive, it is easier; with no support, it can be truly hard. Regarding my brief experience in CoAT, success can easily become failure; it depends on the staff, the community, and of course, your co-therapist.

CoAT work is truly challenging and may not be easy or suitable to others.

As for us – this chapter's writers – we share our experience, and joy, some knowledge, and reflection on the potential and difficulties of school CoAT altogether. We believe that knowledge is power, and we hope that many curious readers will be interested, cautiously experiment and contribute their experiences to the accumulating data on school CoAT.

Notes

1 This term is used here to make a clear distinction between the philosophy and practice of conventional art therapy and CoAT.
2 This term conveys our user-centered approach to therapy, which is distinct from the more conventional, medical approach.
3 CoAT is not utilized in the literature, but rather is used here for the authors' own convenience.
4 "Children" and "students" are used in this chapter interchangeably.
5 For more details, see Ansdell, 2002.
6 Based on Ansdell, (2002).

References

Aigen, K.S. (2014). *The study of music therapy: current issues and concepts*. New York: Routledge.

Animbom Ngong, P. (2017). Theatre: An experience from a mental health clinic in Yaoundé-Cameroon. *Arts & Health: An International Journal for Research, Policy and Practice*, *9*(3). 269–278. doi:10.1080/17533015.2017.1296007

Ansdell, G. (2002). Community music therapy and the winds of change - a discussion paper. In C. Kenny & B. Stige (Eds.), *Contemporary voices in music therapy: Communication, culture and community* (pp.109–143). Oslo: Unipub forlag.

Ansdell, G. (2004). Rethinking music and community: Theoretical perspectives in support of community music therapy. In: M. Pavlicevic & G. Ansdell (Eds.), *Community Music Therapy* (pp. 65–90). Jessica Kingsley Publishers.

Baines, S., Pereira, J., Edwards, J., & Hatch, J. (2019). Queering the curriculum: Why music therapy and other creative arts therapy trainings need queer theory. *Voices: A World Forum for Music Therapy*, *19*(3). https://doi.org/10.15845/voices.v19i3.2676

Belity, I., Regev, D., & Snir, S. (2016). Supervisors' perceptions of art therapy in the Israeli education system. *International Journal of Art Therapy*, *22*(3), 96–105. doi:10.1080/17454832.2016.1245766

Bolger, L., Skews-McFerran, K., & Styge, B. (2018). Hanging out and buying in: Rethinking relationship building to avoid tokenism when striving for collaboration in music therapy. *Music Therapy Perspectives*, *36*(2), 257–266. doi:10.1093/mtp/miy002

Community. (2019). *Dictionary.com*. Retrieved from: https://www.dictionary.com/browse/community?s=t

Davies, A., Richards, E., & Barnwick, N. (2015). *Group music therapy: A group-analytic approach*. London: Routledge.

Elefant, C. (2016). Whose voice is heard? Performances and voices of the Renanim Choir in Israel. In B. Stige, G. Ansdell., C. Elefant, & M. Pavlicevic (Eds.), *Where music helps: Community music therapy in action and reflection* (pp. 189–199). New York: Routledge.

Foulkes, S.H. (1974). My philosophy in psychotherapy. In: E. Foulkes (Ed.), *Selected papers of S.H. Foulkes*. London: Karnac.

Friedman, Y. (1990). *The community school – theory and practice*. Jerusalem: Magness. (In Hebrew).

Harpaz, Y. (2014). *Teaching and learning in a community of thinking: The third model*. New York: Springer.

Huss, E., Kaufman, R., Avgar, A. & Shuker, E. (2016). Arts as a vehicle for community building & post-disaster development. *Disasters 40*(2), 284–303. doi:10.1111/disa.12143.

Inclusive Education (2019). Retrieved from: https://www.unicef.org/education/inclusive-education

Malchiodi, C.A. (2005). Expressive therapies: History, theory, and practice. In C.A. Malchiodi (Ed.), *Expressive therapies* (pp. 1–15). New York: The Guilford Press.

McFerran, K. S., & Rickson, D. (2014). Community music therapy in schools: Realigning with the needs of contemporary students, staff and systems. *International Journal of Community Music*, 7(1), 75–92.

Oliver, M. (2013). The social model of disability: thirty years on. *Disability & Society, 28*(7), 1024–1026. doi:10.1080/09687599.2013.818773

Ottemiller-Drusedum, D., & Awais, Y.J. (2016). A model for art therapists in community-based practice. *Art Therapy*, *33*(3), 144–150. doi:10.1080/07421656.2016.1199245

Pavlicevic, M. (2004). Learning from Thembalethu: Towards responsive and responsible practice in community music therapy. In M. Pavlicevic & G. Ansdell (Eds), *Community music therapy* (pp. 35–48). London: Jessica Kingsley Publishers.

Skews McFerran, K., Thompson, G., & Bolger, L. (2015). The impact of fostering relationships through music within a special school classroom for students with autism spectrum disorder: An action research study. *Educational Action Research*, *24*(2), 241–259. doi:10.1080/09650792.2015.1058171

Snir, S., Regev, D., Keinan, V., Abd El Kader Shahada, H., Salamey, A. Mekel, D., et al., (2018). Art therapy in the Israeli education system – A qualitative meta-analysis. *International Journal of Art Therapy*, *23*(2), 166–167. doi:10.1080/17454832.2017.1409775

Stige, B., Ansdell, G., Elefant, C., & Pavlicevic, M. (2010). *Where music helps: Community music therapy in action and reflection*. Surrey: Ashgate.

Talmor, R., Reiter, S., and Feigin, N. (2004). What about high-burnout education and low-burnout education in the context of integrating students with special needs? *ISER: Issues in Special Education and Rehabilitation*, *19*(1), 17–31. (In Hebrew).

Turner, V. (1969). *Liminality and communitas in the ritual process: Structure and anti-structure*. Chicago: Aldine Publishing.

Zachary, P.N. (2012). Community. In: *Oxford bibliographies*. Retrieved from: https://www.oxfordbibliographies.com/view/document/obo-9780199756384/obo-9780199756384-0080.xml

12 The Role of Art Therapy Substitutes in the Education System during Maternity Leave

Sharon Snir and Racheli Raubach Kaspy

Introduction

There are about 3,500 arts therapists in the Israel education system. Some take maternity leaves that can range from three to six months. Since their employment contracts are similar to those of other teachers and educational staff, the education system is obligated to find a replacement. This procedure, however, is fairly complex.

This chapter is based on a joint study conducted by researchers from the University of Haifa and Tel Hai College. It provides data and insights from interviews with art therapists on issues related to replacing art therapists who go on maternity leave. It discusses the advantages and disadvantages of substitute art therapists and the criteria to take into consideration when making the decision to hire a substitute.

Theoretical Background

Although widespread, temporary replacements for psychotherapists have not received much attention in the literature. Many therapists need to be absent for lengthy periods of time for different reasons such as illness, vacations or maternity leave. During some of these absences, because therapy cannot be halted or postponed for a certain number of clients, the typical solution is to find a replacement (McGourthy, 2013). However, referring clients to a substitute is complex. This is primarily because one of the pillars of psychotherapy is the development of a personal relationship between the therapist and the client (Falkenstrom, Granstrom, & Holmqvist, 2013). For a successful outcome to occur, the therapist and the client must engage in a contract that commits to presence, availability and persistence (Atzil-Slonim et al., 2018; Schwartz, Snir, & Regev, 2018). The ability to create a therapeutic alliance depends on the client's openness and acceptance of the therapeutic relationship as it evolves over the course of therapy (Geller & Porges, 2014). When the therapeutic alliance is stable and strong, it contributes to positive outcomes (Coyne et al., 2017; Koole & Tchacher, 2016) and enables clients to engage in processes of change. From this perspective, a replacement therapist could disrupt the course of therapy (Knowlton, 2018). In case studies in the literature (Chairamonte, 1986; Gibb, 2004; McCarty, Schneider-Braus, & Goodwin, 1986; Sarnat, 1991; Simon, 1992), clinicians report the efforts needed to build a new therapeutic relationship and the clients' need to adjust to the idea of the temporary replacement and build trust. Many clients are concerned that the substitute will not be experienced or understanding, not as sensitive as the original therapist, or not as loving and accepting. In some cases, clients fear that the information conveyed to the replacement may be misinterpreted. In other cases, clients idealize their regular therapist and make comparisons.

When a therapist goes on maternity leave, there are other specific hurdles (McCluskey, 2017; Schmidt, Fiorini, & Ramires, 2015). Pregnancy in general constitutes a challenge to the therapeutic process since the baby is interjected as another actor into the therapeutic space. Clients who perceive the baby as a threat to the therapeutic bond may experience feelings of rivalry and jealousy. Pregnancy, and the impending maternity leave, can also bring abandonment issues to the fore (Korenis & Billick, 2014; Wolfe, 2013). Several authors have raised the concern that certain clients may find it difficult to express their rage and anxiety at the separation from the therapist, which can be coupled with the fear that she may not be able to support these expressions because of her condition (Korenis & Billick, 2014; Wolfe, 2013). The reverse process can also take place when the substitute leaves and the regular therapist returns.

All replacements can trigger stress and anxiety for both the therapist going on leave and the substitute. The therapist going on leave may have to deal with guilt about leaving her clients, which may affect the handover (McCluskey, 2017). Decisions as to the course of therapy are made explicit, which can challenge the therapist's sense of professional adequacy (Raines & Ahlman, 2004). Accordingly, clinicians have noted that the replacement may experience some form of implicit or explicit rivalry with the therapist going on leave (Chairamonte, 1986).

The prime task of the substitute therapist is thus to preserve the continuity of therapy (Schmidt et al., 2015) and the processing of feelings of abandonment related to it (Chairamonte, 1986; McGourty, 2013). The role of the substitute therapist is often conceptualized in the literature as a transitional object or "bridge" who should not develop a therapeutic relationship with the client to avoid disrupting the transference with the original therapist (Lamb & Latona, 1989). Thus, during the replacement period, the substitute serves as a transitional object, a security blanket or a "temporary cure" for the pain created by the departure of the therapist (Sarant, 1991). Both the theoretical and practical literature have put forward several ways to ease the switch in therapists. These include setting a firm date for the replacement and for the return of the therapist, briefing the substitute on the clients' therapeutic history and problems, and arranging a meeting between the substitute, the clients' family and the clinical team. Other recommended steps include arranging for the substitute to meet the clients before the therapist leaves, having a few sessions together (Chairamonte, 1986), providing a transition to sessions with the replacement therapist for a few months before the regular therapist goes on maternity leave (co-therapy) and considering co-therapy after the therapist returns (McCarty et al., 1986).

These recommendations, however, are more complex and may not be feasible when art therapy is provided in the school system, since the integration of art therapy in the educational system in general has its own specific hurdles. These hurdles include difficulties resulting from the combination of the therapeutic and the educational cultures, which have different languages, different goals and at times perceived conflicts of interests (Snir et al., 2018). Kaspy Raubach (Raubach Kaspy, Snir, Regev, & Harpazy, 2020) studied the perceptions of substitutes, art therapists on maternity leave, supervisors and school counselors who accompanied the substitute during this time period with respect to the replacement process. This study led to the founding of a discussion group made up of leading art therapist supervisors in the education system in Israel. As part of this discussion group, a survey was sent to all supervisors and art therapists in the education system who had been involved in maternity leave replacements in schools and kindergartens. The survey was completed by 73 respondents who described the best ways, based on their own experiences, to deal with substitution. This chapter describes the reality of the replacement of art therapists who go on a maternity leave in Israel, based upon the Kaspy-Raubach study, the discussion group and the survey findings, and suggests a model for optimal implementation of the replacement process.

Description of the Working Model and Clinical Examples

Systemic Challenges

Many respondents signaled the importance of finding a replacement for students when their therapist goes on maternity leave. They cited the importance of the continuity of therapy, the students' right to therapy and the possibilities of achieving new therapeutic targets with a substitute therapist. Schools have a budget for art therapy positions, which is available when a therapist goes on maternity leave, and schools want to use it because otherwise this funding is lost. Nevertheless, the findings emerging from the Kaspy-Raubach study and the focus group suggested that the replacement of art therapists in the education system is a challenging process. This challenge is intensified because of the differences in the perception of the role of the substitute between the therapeutic language and the educational language. However, the Ministry of Education views art therapists as employees and considers their replacement to be the equivalent of finding a substitute for any other teacher.

This difference in concerns between therapist and the school system is manifested in the lack of specific handover procedures. The current guidelines for arts therapists in the Israeli education system do not address ways to integrate substitute art therapists. The Ministry of Education considers that the handover is not part of the substitute's job profile, and does not finance on-the-job training hours. However, there is an implicit expectation that the handover will take place on the substitute's own time. Since the Ministry of Education does not compensate the handover, this creates a situation where the substitute can only see the clients and get information about them, get paid and be covered by insurance when the therapist has already left for maternity leave. The supervisors noted in the interviews that for this reason, they cannot hire a substitute art therapist in advance, and they need to wait for the last moment. The last moment may be difficult to anticipate since the date of birth is often uncertain in itself. In addition, despite wanting a smooth transition, maternity leave may start earlier than planned. Similarly, the return of the art therapist is not pre-determined. According to Ministry of Education guidelines, the therapist is not obligated to define a specific return date. Thus, therapists may extend or cut back on their leaves of absence at short notice, which makes the end of the replacement unexpected.

The administrative process of hiring arts therapists can also present challenges. In situations where the substitute is not already on the Ministry of Education payroll, hiring can be a lengthy process involving confirmations and certifications. The bureaucratic red tape contributes to the uncertainty about their position and can lead to confusion that delays the handover process.

Finding an available substitute is also more complicated when the school is interested in a replacement for the same time slots as the therapist on maternity leave. The substitute cannot always work in the time frame of the therapist on leave. This means changing students' therapy hours, the classes that they will miss while in therapy and making sure the therapy room is available at new times, which can cause conflicts among the different actors involved in the replacement.

Despite these problems, many new therapists consider substitution as a good opportunity to be hired by the Ministry of Education since it can improve their chances of getting a permanent position as an arts therapist. For the system, substitution is an opportunity to test the capabilities of the substitute to deal with the challenges of the job (Raubach-Kaspy et al., submitted).

The Handover

Given the lack of budget and guidelines, the handover rarely takes place smoothly and its success depends on the readiness and goodwill of the substitute and the departing therapist. Typically, the handover takes place close to term, when the therapist is busy writing reports, therapy summaries, organizing farewells with the clients and holding summary sessions with the parents. The departing therapist may also not be fully mentally available in this period so close to the birth, and often the replacement has no contact with the departing therapist before she leaves. At other times, when the school interviews several candidates, the departing therapist must meet with each of them, and repeatedly provide information on the clients, while making sure to avoid breaching confidentiality. The actual handover may be brief, and not be sufficient for the therapist to transfer enough information about the clients or allow the substitute to get acquainted with the educational environment and staff. This results in situations where the substitute has to deal by him/herself with technical issues such as finding the location of the therapy room, adapting the therapy space to his/her arts modality and dealing with a lack of supplies of art materials. In such cases of poor handover, the substitute may not always have a good grasp of the school's point of view, and the staff sometimes finds it difficult to understand the substitute's point of view. This misunderstanding can result in miscommunication and may sometimes undermine the replacement. The lack of sufficient overlap and the transfer of partial information about the client make it difficult for the substitute to understand the departing therapist's approaches to separation and the clients' responses to the separation. This lack of information makes it difficult to select the optimal form of therapy for each client.

The interviews suggested that the departing therapists transferred client information in different ways to the substitutes. In cases where a substitute has not yet been found, some therapists transfer information about the clients to a third party to make sure that the information reaches the substitute. Some therapists leave reports about their clients with the school system, while others add personal notes. Sometimes the entire handover process takes place by phone. Certain participants emphasized the need to review the basic work procedures, especially when the substitute was new to the educational framework, since a telephone handover was not sufficient to discuss the clients in depth. In some cases, the supervisors acted as the go-between for the substitutes and the department that assigns therapists to schools. The supervisors said that it is often difficult to find the right person in the school who can help, and that the substitutes' integration depended to a great extent on the team culture.

A lack of familiarity with the educational system during the handover can make it difficult for substitute therapists to understand basic issues such as how to schedule their working hours, how to write reports and how to integrate themselves with the teaching staff. The interviews suggested that substitutes do not always get the help they need from the system, but, in cases where this did take place, the involvement of supervisors helped ease the transition.

The supervisors oversee the replacement process and cope with the needs of the school system, the substitute and the therapist on leave. Some stated that they had to "walk on thin ice" to accommodate the system's demands with the principles of art therapy. In some cases, they personally introduced the substitute to the educational staff. Supervisors mentioned situations where they helped the substitute devise a therapy plan for each educational framework. When they were not available to help the substitute during the handover, they organized personal supervision hours. As part of their job they accompany the substitutes in their work, and figure out solutions, while trying to process challenging and conflicting issues during the replacement.

Educational counselors also play an important role in the replacement process. The educational counselors function in some cases as an intermediary who helps coordinate the therapy schedule, reserve therapy rooms and define the nature of therapy. In cases where there is no handover, these educational counselors are the link between the substitutes, the homeroom teachers and the clients. They introduce substitutes to the homeroom teachers, tell the clients that a substitute is coming and get them ready for her/his arrival. Some counselors stated that they played an active role in setting up the initial contact between the therapist and the clients, and by taking them to the therapy room. Occasionally they made sure that the substitute was invited to staff meetings to get background information on the clients. In cases where the team was not open to accepting substitutes, some of the counselors reported that they contributed to efforts to integrate the substitute within the team. As part of their efforts, they deal with situations where the fit is positive and the substitute is experienced as contributing, but also with situations where the "temporary guest" wants to change existing working habits, which can cause conflicts. The counselors reported that they were expected to hold, contain and support the substitute, while at times dealing with their own workload, especially when there were severe problems with students. These tended to take precedence over the substitute's well-being.

Challenges During the Replacement

One of the key dilemmas created by substitution has to do with the essence of therapy itself: should the therapy provided by the substitute be defined as a new therapy or the continuation of the previous therapy? This dilemma also captures the conflict in interests between the goals of the school system, which is interested in simply maintaining the provision of therapy with minimal changes, and the therapeutic view which considers each case as separate and unique, that requires re-thinking and re-organization, and therefore also a period of familiarization that enables a new therapeutic alliance with the client to form. This dilemma is also related to the issue of which therapeutic goals are worthwhile to work on during the replacement period. The short period of time allocated to the substitute also means that he or she must decide on priorities when fixing the goal of therapy for each client. In addition, given the availability of therapists for brief periods of replacement work, it may not always be possible to find a therapist with the same modality as the therapist on leave. While a change in modality (for example, from an art therapist to a drama therapist) may be viewed in certain situations as positive in that it helps differentiate the two therapists, when the substitute's specialization does not fit the clients' needs, and/or when the therapist works in a setting that is not adapted to his or her own modality, there can be actual damage to the ongoing therapeutic climate and outcomes.

Other professional dilemmas center on issues of separation from the regular therapist, but also separation from the substitute upon her return. The theoretical and research literature describe the ethical and practical importance of clients' identification that is suitable for short-term therapy, as occurs in the process of replacement (Abbass, Rabung, Leichsenring, Refseth, & Midgley, 2013). The substitute therapists interviewed for this study (Raubach Kaspy et al., submitted) mentioned their fears that short-term therapies may bring back traumas from the client's past, as described in the literature (Knafo, 2018; Lam, 2017), and that the absence of expectations and clarifications between the therapists, the client and the school can engender situations where the impact of the replacement on the clients is not given sufficient attention. These difficulties may be intensified by the difficulty of planning the separation process when the replacement time frame is unknown and can vary since some therapists return early from maternity leave.

One of the challenges the substitute faces is creating a network of relationships with the educational staff. Some substitutes said that they were subject to constant comparison with the regular therapist. Some said that they were forced to justify their approach to therapy and explain that each art therapist uses his or her own style and works in a different way, which means that treatments will differ. The substitutes talked about tensions when the educational staff did not support them in cases where their approach differed from that of the regular therapist. For example, a therapist said that she was criticized by the staff for choosing to intervene using art materials, and not continue to work with the regular therapist's puppet theater technique. This lack of understanding and support on the part of the educational teams were also manifested in other situations. For example, a substitute described an instance where she was working with a group of students with Attention Deficit Disorder, and the educational team that was present in the room simply started to chat about personal issues and interrupted during the therapeutic session. Some of the substitutes noted that because they are new to the system and want to make a good impression without getting into clashes with the staff, they do not comment in situations such as these. Others said that they did not try to change ongoing treatments and carried out the staff's requests even though they thought that switching from group therapy to individual therapy, or providing other intervention, would actually be better for the clients. Sometimes the staff considered that the artworks simply took up space and suggested throwing away some and letting the students take the rest home. Others said that sometimes there was no place for them to raise their professional concerns. In some situations, the educational staff expected the substitutes to do tasks that exceeded their role as arts therapists. They said that the system sometimes takes advantage of the confusion during replacement by allocating clients to therapy who are not eligible, by capitalizing on the substitute's desire to be accepted by the system. The lack of understanding of the educational staff, in some cases, leads to difficulties in managing the replacement. There were even cases where the school assigned an art teacher rather than an arts therapist because they saw no difference between the two (Raubach Kaspy et al., submitted).

Difficulties that are familiar to therapists who work in the education system, such as the lack of art materials, the shortage of musical instruments, a room that is not suitable for therapy, treatment conducted outdoors under less than optimal conditions for art making, and staff who enter in the room in the middle of the session and do not respect the students' privacy (Moriya, 2006; Snir et al.,2018) were described in the study (Raubach Kaspy et al., submitted) as intensified in the case of substitutes, who are sometimes forced to compromise their therapeutic standards in the face of a system that sees them as a temporary "band-aid." Some described situations where there was not enough storage space and the artworks were exposed elsewhere, not in the therapy room. The participants mentioned the lack of clarity with respect to preserving artworks made with the therapist who went on maternity leave: What should be done with them? Should they be kept? Thrown away? How should substitutes cope with situations in which the therapy room was cleared without letting them know and in which sometimes the clients were even present when their works were thrown into the garbage?

The interviews conducted during this study showed that there are situations in which the substitutes are part of a system that is pushing them to start working to avoid a break in the continuity of therapy, whereas they are legally obligated to wait for parents' renewed consent. During the wait, the substitute is sometimes asked to start therapy without reading any reports, observation of the students or meeting with the parents for intake. Some substitutes said that during the replacement period, they were unsure whether to report client-related issues because of the short period of acquaintance with the students and their parents. Others described a situation in which at the end of their role as substitutes, they had to leave the therapy to a third party because they could not accompany the case themselves.

Some substitutes reported that they had difficulties with students who wanted to wait for the former therapist to return, and had problems establishing a relationship with the new therapist. Some mentioned the clients' silence during the therapy hour or their reluctance to cooperate. Supervisors said that they had faced a dilemma as to the replacement's viability in cases in which the replacement created difficulties with clients. In addition, there were counselors who noted that the school system is obligated to provide therapy on a regular basis, and does so without at times considering all the consequences for individual students. Both substitutes and outgoing therapists noted that for clients who have problems adjusting to changes and have abandonment issues, a replacement for a short period of three months may result in emotional difficulties. Certain substitutes mentioned that the students are not asked whether they would prefer to wait for the therapist on leave to return.

The Experiences of the Professionals Involved in the Replacement Process

The therapists going on leave said they experienced the excitement and fears related to the impending birth alongside feelings of guilt about leaving their clients in the middle of the therapy process. In cases where the baby was premature, and they were not able to separate properly and prepare the clients for the replacement, their feelings of guilt were intensified. Some of them described pregnancy and separation as an overwhelming experience for them because of the students' reactions to the pregnancy that ranged from wonder, joy and sometimes even anger to disregard, "acting-out" and abandonment anxiety. Some said that the separation with clients who had been in therapy for several years was difficult for them especially because these clients needed to deal with the fact that the therapist had a personal life outside the framework of therapy. The therapists going on leave said that finding a substitute gave them a feeling of relief since despite the problems their clients would have the opportunity to continue therapy. They said that they felt responsibility and concern for their clients and were relieved when a substitute was found that could be trusted. On the other hand, some departing therapists mentioned feelings of jealousy and rivalry arising from comparisons that can arise between them and the substitute. Sometimes this was also accompanied by feelings of fear and uncertainty that stemmed from not knowing whether they would return to the school where they worked. They expressed fear of a situation in which the substitute would be so successful that she would remain beyond the replacement period and they would be transferred to another framework.

The substitutes described their mixed emotions in relation to the replacement. They said they were able to experience it from a mature place where they were aware of the essence of the process, but sometimes experienced strong emotions such as treason, abandonment and exploitation. In contrast to clinicians who define the role of the substitute as a "bridge" or a transitional object (Lamb & Latona, 1989), some of the substitutes described feelings of frustration at being "a filler" or a "band aid" in the educational system which was "disposed of" when the system finished using it. They claimed that because of their awareness of the replacement process, its transient nature and the fact that they were new to the system, they could relate to it in a conscious manner, while another side of them also experienced powerful emotional reactions to the complex situation of the replacement. The substitutes described their feelings of loneliness, especially when the replacement was for a short period of time. Some said they felt frustrated by the fact that there were no built-in accompanying mechanisms or supervision to help them start in the educational system. This frustration strengthened their feeling of helplessness, given the expectations placed on them to integrate quickly on the job. This made them feel that they were not sufficiently appreciated in relation to their level of investment and devotion. The complex meetings with the staff, comparisons with the outgoing therapist and the challenges in creating relationship with the clients were described by some of the participants as a shock to their self-image. Ending the replacement raised various and varied feelings in each of the substitutes. Some described the disappointment they experienced when they discovered that the salary was very low, which enhanced the sense of exploitation. Others described their uncertainty about not knowing whether they would continue working at the school or would even continue to be employed by the therapeutic center. There were substitutes who said they felt satisfaction when the staff acknowledged their work and gave them positive feedback, and others said the system and the staff wanted them to stay and they felt pride in having been able to cope with all the challenges of the replacement, although this sense of satisfaction was mixed with a feeling of guilt that they might take the work of the therapists on leave. There were substitutes who described the separation from the clients as an overwhelming experience accompanied by concern for clients who had formed a deep therapeutic alliance. Substitutes who already had experience with replacement described themselves as ready for the separation process while reminding the clients that the former therapist would soon be back from her maternity leave. In addition to all that was said, the substitutes described the work with the clients as a source of great satisfaction and said that when the door closed in the art therapy room, all their frustrations were left behind, especially when beneficial relationships were created with the clients and they experienced significant advances in therapy. Some of them felt the satisfaction of being a "good enough mother" who is doing everything she can to allow these children a safe and contained place that helps them not to feel the lack of the therapists going on leave.

When Is It Appropriate to Recruit a Substitute and When Is It Not?

All the participants in the interviews, the focus group and the survey agreed that replacement should not take place automatically, and that several key issues should be considered before assigning a substitute. One consistent argument was that it is important to have a replacement in situations where there are mental and/or functional difficulties that make it impossible to leave the students without a therapeutic solution. Both from the students' and from the system's points of view, replacement is more meaningful, and inspires confidence and a feeling of "I will not be left alone," when it lasts longer (here the opinions were divided; some suggested it should last more than three months, and others mentioned only in the event of maternity leave of over six months) and takes place sequentially without intervening vacations. Replacement in the last few months of the year (some argued in the second half of the year) can cause more damage than good, and can elicit a feeling of abandonment. Similarly, a replacement for a month or two at the beginning of the year was also perceived as not effective. Some claimed that in cases of individual therapy, especially when establishing a therapeutic alliance is difficult, as with Autism Spectrum Disorder students, it is preferable not to have a replacement, but to take advantage of the time to hire another health professional to strengthen another area – for example, occupational therapy or academic proficiency in accordance with the needs of the client.

Even after the decision has been made to hire a substitute, each student should be considered separately to determine whether he or she would benefit from a substitute. According to some of the participants, younger students may benefit more from the replacement, since older students may have more problems creating a bond when they know it is temporary, since they are already able to form more profound and meaningful relationships. At the same time, there are students who may have already worked with several therapists, for whom a break from therapy may be beneficial as a period of coping without a therapist. There may be cases in which students are not interested in the replacement, or parents who relinquish this right, because they decide that their child would not benefit from the replacement, and in such cases they can request other forms of support.

Even when all other conditions are met, it remains unclear whether the substitute will be accepted well. Is there a team to support the replacement? Are the teachers available to mediate and support the replacement? Does the substitute's schedule comply with the needs of the school?

Principles of Substitute Selection

In terms of the factors that contribute to the replacement and associated with the substitute her/himself, the experienced substitutes who had previously participated in replacements were aware and experienced with the challenges involved in short therapy and the implications it has on the clients. Since senior therapists are more experienced, some suggested establishing a "substitutes pool" to be available for replacement. Others argued that young therapists can also be mature enough to be successful substitutes. Motivation is also very important in the ability to cope with the challenges. Therefore, seniority was not considered a pre-condition, but maturity, self-confidence and the ability to develop contacts were felt to be important in coping with rejection, anger and the objections of clients to changes related to replacement.

Some of the interviewees related to the therapist's personality as an essential factor for the success of the replacement. They described several personal features of a substitute that help to do his/her job and integrate successfully into the system that included modesty, seriousness and responsibility. They also noted certain capabilities and skills that help deal with the complexity of the role, such as the ability to compromise and flexibility. Supervisors mentioned it is important that the substitute should "put his/her ego aside," have the flexibility to adapt or match what is common at school and the ways of working of the previous therapist, even if it is not his or her most natural way. The supervisors suggested that the substitutes should have the capacity to contain a good ability to communicate with the staff and to work as part of a team. It is important for them to accept that their role is temporary, realize what it means and how to help students accept the change and the separations associated with it.

Substitutes should be familiar with models of short-term therapy. The substitute should be able to specify the nature of the therapeutic contract. The substitute therapists said that knowing the procedures and methods in the education system is a challenge itself, which adds more confusion and an extra burden to the challenges of replacement. Substitutes should thus be familiar with the workings of the school system. Familiarity and experience with similar populations is important, as well as the motivation to work with the students and an understanding of the specific features of this population. Finally, there are many advantages to having a substitute who is part of the school's therapeutic team in terms of the familiarity with the system and the students.

Some participants supported the idea of hiring a substitute who has the same modality since it creates continuity and also increases the likelihood of having a suitable room. By contrast, some argued that the change in modality should not be a problem, and can even be beneficial in emphasizing the transition, the difference between the two therapies and increasing openness to the differences between the therapists. In the end, the decision depends on the reality at the school, and the availability and the schedule of the replacement.

One of the difficulties that came up in the study relates to the fact that substitutes are working in several schools at the same time. Therefore, it is recommended that the substitute should work a part-time job and at not more than one-third to half of a full-time job, while attempting not to split his/her job between too many institutions. Since many therapists who are working in the education system in Israel are assigned to several different schools, the therapists who go on maternity leave need to be replaced by more than one substitute therapist. Similarly, Regev, Green-Orlovich and Snir (2015) found that when the therapist's job is split between several schools, it affects the amount of time he or she can spend in one educational framework, and consequently, the way each school is able to collaborate. This situation may account for the weak system commitment to therapists and therapy needs. This situation becomes more complex and intensified during a short replacement period.

Recommendation for the Handover

The therapists and the supervisors who participated in the interviews in the focus group and in the survey said that it is impossible to offer a unified and structured picture of replacement since there is a great deal of difference in the needs and possibilities of all the parties involved, and it is important to take everyone into account when planning the replacement. Therefore, an open dialogue, the coordination of expectations and the agreement of all those involved is essential for an effective replacement. For these reasons, the following recommendations constitute thinking points and refer to cases of planning and finding a substitute for an art therapist going on maternity leave.

The substitute search process should start as early as in the last trimester of pregnancy. The process may be long, so it is better not to wait until the last moment. It is important to devote time for the outgoing therapist and for the substitute to manage the handover. Most of the survey respondents and most of the interviewees said that the Ministry of Education needs to allocate resources to pay for the handover, and that adequate monetary compensation would contribute to enabling the handover to take place in a methodical and professional manner. The views on the ideal handover time varied from two hours to two weeks. The participants agreed that the supervisor should accompany the process, and should support the handover fully in a professional manner by transferring the information, defining the schedule, helping with integrating at school, setting goals and objectives and ensuring that a suitable therapy room is available. That said, the handover should meet the needs of the substitute therapist, and it is important to listen to what s/he needs and what is important for him or her to adapt to the position.

To facilitate the entry of the substitute, and for his/her adaptation to the system to be as smooth as possible, the departing therapist should introduce the replacement to the school staff, the therapy room and the workplace. In getting to know the staff, the departing therapist should make it clear how the substitute can be helped by the staff, and which issues are not worth pursuing. All the research and survey participants stressed the importance of a joint meeting between both therapists, the educational team, the teachers and the school counselor to formulate a work plan that suits the clients. The planning should also include the question of which clients should continue therapy with the substitute. There may be clients with whom there was a significant relationship, or a process that ended, and there is no need to continue. Furthermore, it is important for professionals treating the student outside of school, such as the psychiatrist or welfare services, to be informed. In preparing the therapy room, it is important to help the replacement prepare it for his/her needs, order missing equipment and organize the room in a way that is right for him/her. If this is done together, before the therapist goes on maternity leave, the therapist's feelings when she returns may be ameliorated.

The research and survey participants recommended that the therapists going on leave should prepare a folder (or a computerized secured file) with her own set of hours and data on each student, including the main themes in therapy and sensitive points that are important to know. In cases where the therapist going on leave is handing over a group to the substitute, it is important to convey information regarding the work that was done, the characteristics of the group, processes that have taken place, the objectives of the therapy and the interpersonal relationships within the group. It is important to supply information about the characteristics of work with the parents, their cooperation, the way of working with them so far and recommendations about how to continue. The folder should include the educational plan for each student, in an organized manner, and a summary of therapy and reports. The conversation between the outgoing and the incoming therapists should also include the departing therapist's perceptions of the ongoing goals and the modes of intervention. In addition, the departing therapists should specify their availability for additional inquiries if necessary during the replacement.

The Recommended Procedures for the Parties Involved in Relation to Preparation of the Educational Framework

Among the substitutes interviewed for the study (Raubach Kaspy et al., submitted), some noted that one of the factors helping substitutes is the educational team's willingness to accept them. They said that when the team took responsibility and created a personal and professional relationship with them, they felt they belonged and were wanted to a greater extent, which contributed to their adjustment to the system. Certain substitutes said that the collaboration with the staff and discussing the clients in regular team meetings was a significant factor in the success of the replacement. The therapists who responded to the survey said that it was important to make sure whether the teams are ready to accept a substitute, and are interested in his or her entry into the school system, before the decision is made to hire a substitute. From their experience, there are situations in which the staff is not available, and in such situations it is preferable not to engage in a replacement process in the first place. If the decision is made to hire a substitute, it is important to prepare the educational staff for his/her arrival so that they can be more responsive to his or her needs and be cooperative. During the preparation stage, a discussion about how the substitute will join the team socially and personally may contribute to more productive teamwork. It is also important to show the substitutes the way the school is run, and at the same time explain to the team its role in supporting substitute therapy, for example, by maintaining regular therapy hours and maintaining the clients' privacy during the session. It is important for the therapist going on leave to prepare the team and to listen to the voices and experiences of this discourse. To encourage the team to help make the replacement process successful, it is important to share thinking about the process and to allow shared ideas to emerge. The staff needs to define their needs within the school framework, both for themselves and for the substitute. This will be the basis for coordinating expectations between the system and the substitute. Educational teams in the school need to be involved in thinking and making decisions about which clients will continue with the substitute, and about the therapy goals. It is important to appoint one member of the team as a contact person for the substitute to help him or her deal with school issues and in organizing the space and the therapy room. Naturally, the school must have a room ready that is appropriate for the substitute therapist or help him/her to re-arrange the current room for therapy. The educational team should be made aware of the importance of integration of the substitute therapist, even if for a short period of time, and their significant role in his/her ability to do his or her best. It is important to remind the educational staff to invite the substitute to their meetings, maintain a continuous dialogue and address requests and inquiries.

How Should Students Be Prepared for the Replacement?

As stated above, the discourse with the students and preparing them for the replacement must take into account their age, their difficulties, their ability to accept a change and express themselves. In any case, since the replacement can bring up issues of connection, trust, abandonment and change, it is important to make preparations for the replacement. This preparation should include discussing the therapist's departure on maternity leave and an explanation of what can be expected when the substitute arrives. It should also include information about the duration of the replacement, when the therapist going on leave is planning to return and whether there will be a change in the modality and the form of therapy (for example, transitioning from individual therapy to group therapy). In the discourse with the clients, it is important to invite them to express their feelings about the replacement. Certain clients may oppose replacement, and some of the survey respondents argued that it is important to find out what the clients want and allow them to refuse. It is important to legitimize the emotions that may arise but also to emphasize the importance of the replacement and the opportunities that it provides for a new relationship, the wonderful possibility of meeting another therapist, and another creative mode of treatment, an opportunity to see things from a new perspective and to create change. Many participants in the study suggested having a joint meeting between the student and the therapists going on leave and the substitute. Similar recommendations were suggested by clinicians, who saw the pre-therapy sessions with the therapist going on leave and the substitute as an opportunity to prepare the clients for the transition (Chairamonte, 1986; Gibb, 2004; McCarty et al., 1986; Sarnat, 1991). This type of meeting can convey the mutual confidence of the therapists in each other to the student, together with the feeling that he or she is being contained and protected by them together. It can help clients accept the change. At this type of meeting, the therapeutic goals and the changing setting can be defined together. Even towards the end of the replacement period, it is important to have another meeting between the outgoing and the incoming therapists, for purposes of sequencing and continuity, and a redefinition of the goals and the setting.

How Should the Parents Be Prepared for the Replacement?

It is advisable to meet with the parents in advance to discuss what will take place when the therapist leaves and for how long, as well as informing them who is going to replace her. It is important for the parents to hear about the replacement from the therapist going on leave, and not from the student, since parents may feel anxious about the expected change. If possible, it is important for the parents to be partners in the thinking process about the replacement for their child, the expected benefits and the possible costs, in a way that will enable them to take part in the decision of whether and how the replacement will unfold. It is also a good time for the parents to look back to see what their child and themselves have accomplished so far, and to think about what they would like to do in the future. The purpose of the discussion is not only knowledge, but also to obtain parental consent, and even invite them to take part in the process, as this alliance will also be passed on to their child. It is worth engaging the parents in a discussion of ways they can support the process, and how they can mediate the transition. It can reduce the parents' anxiety and help them get used to the change and mediate the transition to their child. If possible, the therapist going on leave should introduce the substitute to the parents. This provides an opportunity to discuss the way the substitute will work with their child, define goals together, and examine the setting and its suitability for the student. The parents should be informed about the new therapy plan, and if therapy will take place in a new modality that they are unfamiliar with, it should be explained as well. The parents need to hear about how they can get in touch with the substitute so that they feel they have someone to talk to, despite the fact that the therapist is going on leave. In the conversation, the transition and the separation from the departing therapist should be connected to the contents from the student's therapeutic process.

What Important Principles Should the Substitute Implement During the Replacement Period?

The replacement period may involve reactions by the clients to the departure of the therapist. Therefore, during the replacement period there should be a place for expressing emotions such as jealousy, abandonment and perhaps detachment that can arise. The substitute can help elaborate the meaningful relationship with the former therapist by connecting between what took place, what is being experienced and the future. At the practical level, in the interviews the therapists described the ways in which they contained the passage of time for the clients. For example, some therapists made a train with carriages that symbolized the passing weeks. In addition to suggesting to the substitutes to create a continuum and continuity by referring to the regular therapist's goals and interventions, the survey participants also recommended having a clear perception that the therapy in the replacement is not the same as the previous one, but rather a new, complementary, time-limited treatment.

As stated above, many participants in the broader study stated that the replacement, whose therapeutic intervention is limited in time, should be based on the principles of short-term treatment, focused on pre-defined goals, the issue of separation or in establishing a relationship. Sometimes the treatment will be pre-defined as maintenance care alone. At times, it is possible to maintain focused group therapy on subjects such as strengthening social skills or another structured purpose. The participants argued that it is important that the substitute be given an opportunity for the new relationship to evolve, discuss the opportunity for something new and get other points of view.

Finally, it is important that the substitutes have a commitment to get supervision and make sure that they have someone in school to consult with in case of need. It is advisable to have intense supervision especially in cases of therapists who are new to the educational system. In addition, the substitute should take part in a supervision group. It is crucial for the substitute to be assisted when he or she begins in the educational system, the new school, planning his/her therapeutic goals and when deciding on the choice of interventions. The supervision should also include technical and institutional integration to help in thinking about developing therapeutic programs and what is right or wrong in this framework. Some argued that there is no difference between a substitute and other arts therapists, but the majority noted that there is a need for a unique approach, and providing more assistance than usual for the substitutes.

The decision on an appropriate model to work with depends on the professional perceptions of the people involved. It is dependent on the substitute's training and his/her familiarity with treatment methods. It is of course related to the needs of the clients and the system's perception of these needs. Many survey respondents said that sometimes when the art therapist is going on maternity leave, the role of the substitute can be maintenance and emotional support until the therapist returns. Many suggested that continuation of individual therapy during brief periods of substitution may increase the feeling of abandonment, and in some situations, it is preferable for some of the clients to be offered group therapy instead. Many participants conceptualized the replacement period as a time-limited therapy and suggested that thinking about the replacement period as a short-term treatment and about appropriate objectives and interventions is the most appropriate when coping with the challenges involved in replacement. There were many proposals for working in a structured model (some of these models are described in other chapters in this book) that can include the class as a group, open studio, Group Theater, musical composition and psychoeducational projects. Some suggested that the replacement period can be a time to experience a focused therapy technique, such as Cognitive Behavioral methods, Mindfulness or more targeted goals such as improving social skills, development of playfulness or increased emotional regulation, depending on the substitute's specialization and training.

Summary and Conclusions

The integration of the arts therapy profession in educational settings has expanded in recent years. Many key questions have been raised as to how to best integrate it so that it does not undermine the therapeutic essence while still allowing arts therapists to treat students under the appropriate conditions. Much effort has been made to address the difficulties that arise during the replacement period to develop an effective model that responds to situations when the therapist goes on maternity leave.

The challenges described in this chapter characterize the education system in Israel. At the same time, this model can form the basis for thinking about the process of replacing arts therapists in education systems in other countries. The online possibilities that therapists are now implementing during the COVID crisis may be adapted as ways to conduct the handover even under the conditions and limitations described in this chapter.

Acknowledgments

We would like to thank all the interviewees, who so willingly contributed their experience and knowledge. We are grateful to Israel Department of Education national arts therapist supervisors (at the time of this writing) Anat Marnin-Shaham and Anat Mendelson for initiating this research, taking part in the interviews and for partnering us to advance this study. Special thanks go to Efrat Roginsky, Zvia Cohen, Miki Mentch, Shlomit Seri and Hamutal Amit for taking part in the focus group, the survey construction, and in reviewing this paper.

References

Abbass, A.A., Rabung, S., Leichsenring, F., Refseth, J.S., & Midgley, N. (2013). Psychodynamic psychotherapy for children and adolescents: A meta-analysis of short-term psychodynamic models. *Journal of the American Academy of Child & Adolescent Psychiatry*, *52*(8), 863–875.

Atzil-Slonim, D., Bar-Kalifa, E., Fisher, H., Peri, T., Lutz, W., Rubel, J., & Rafaeli, E. (2018). Emotional congruence between clients and therapists and its effect on treatment outcome. *Journal of Counseling Psychology*, *65*(1), 51.

Chiaramonte, J.A. (1986). Therapist pregnancy and maternity leave: Maintaining and furthering therapeutic gains in the interim. *Clinical Social Work Journal*, *14*(4), 335–348.

Coyne, A. E., Constantino, M. J., Laws, H. B., Westra, H. A., & Antony, M. M. (2017). Patient–therapist convergence in alliance ratings as a predictor of outcome in psychotherapy for generalized anxiety disorder. *Psychotherapy Research*, 1–16. Online First Publication. https://doi. org/10.1080/10503307.2017.1303209

Falkenström, F., Granström, F., & Holmqvist, R. (2013). Therapeutic alliance predicts symptomatic improvement session by session. *Journal of Counseling Psychology*, *60*(3), 317.

Geller, S.M., & Porges, S.W. (2014). Therapeutic presence: Neurophysiological mechanisms mediating feeling safe in therapeutic relationships. *Journal of Psychotherapy Integration*, *24*(3), 178.

Gibb, D.E. (2004). Reliving abandonment in the face of the therapist's pregnancy. *Psychoanalytic Psychotherapy*, *18*(1), 67–85.

Knafo, D. (2018). Beginnings and endings: Time and termination in psychoanalysis. *Psychoanalytic Psychology*, *35*(1), 8.

Knowlton, G.G. (2018). *Anticipated therapist absences: The therapist's lens*. (Unpublished doctoral dissertation). Marquette University. Retrieved from: https://epublications.marquette.edu/dissertations_mu/785

Koole, S.L., & Tschacher, W. (2016). Synchrony in psychotherapy: A review and an integrative framework for the therapeutic alliance. *Frontiers in Psychology*, 7, 862.

Korenis, P., & Billick, S.B. (2014). The pregnant therapist: The effect of a negative pregnancy outcome on a psychotherapy patient. *Psychiatric Quarterly*, *85*(3), 377–382.

Lam, W.I. (2017). *The time to say goodbye: Lived experience of forced termination from a drama therapy perspective.* Retrieved from: https://spectrum.library.concordia.ca/982561/

Lamb, D.H., & Latona, J.R. (1989). The substitute therapist as transitional object in the treatment of borderline personality disorders. *Psychotherapy: Theory, Research, Practice, Training*, *26*(3), 323–329.

McCarty, T., Schneider-Braus, K., & Goodwin, J. (1986). Use of alternate therapist during pregnancy leave. *The Journal of the American Academy of Psychoanalysis*, *14*(3), 377–383.

McCluskey, M. (2017). The pregnant therapist: A qualitative examination of the client experience. *Clinical Social Work Journal*, *45*(4), 301–310.

McGourty, A. (2013). The pregnant therapist and the psychotic client: A phenomenological understanding of the impact of the therapist's pregnancy on the therapeutic process. *European Journal of Psychotherapy & Counselling*, *15*(1), 18–31.

Moriya, D. (2006). Ethical issues in school art therapy. *Art Therapy*, *23*(2), 59–65.

Raines, J.C., & Ahlman, C. (2004). No substitute for competence: How to survive and thrive as an interim school social worker. *School Social Work Journal*, *28*(2), 37–52.

Raubach Kaspy, R., Snir, S., Regev, D., & Harpazy, S. (2020). *Art therapists', supervisors' and school counselors' perceptions of the substitute art therapist's role in the education system during maternity leave*. Manuscript submitted for publication.

Regev, D., Green-Orlovich, A., & Snir, S. (2015). Art therapy in schools–The therapist's perspective. *The Arts in Psychotherapy*, *45*, 47–55.

Sarnat, J.E. (1991). When a therapist goes on leave. *Psychotherapy: Theory, Research, Practice, Training*, *28*(4), 650–659. doi:10.1037/0033-3204.28.4.650

Schmidt, F.M.D., Fiorini, G.P., & Röhnelt Ramires, V.R. (2015). Psychoanalytic psychotherapy and the pregnant therapist: A literature review. Research in Psychotherapy: Psychopathology. *Process and Outcome*, 18(2), 50–61. doi: 10.4081/ripppo.2015.185

Schwarz, N., Snir, S., & Regev, D. (2018). The therapeutic presence of the art therapist. *Art Therapy*, *35*(1), 11–18.

Simon, J.C. (1992). The group therapist's absence and the substitute leader. *International Journal of Group Psychotherapy*, *42*(2), 287–291.

Snir, S., Regev, D., Keinan, V., Abd El Kader-Shahada, H., Salamey, A., Mekel, D.,… Alkara, M. (2018). Art therapy in the Israeli education system–a qualitative meta-analysis. *International Journal of Art Therapy*, *23*(4), 169–179.

Wolfe, E.H. (2013). *The therapist's pregnancy and the client-therapist relationship: An exploratory study*. Doctoral Dissertation, Smith College School for Social Work.

Index

For Product Safety Concerns and Information please contact our EU representative GPSR@taylorandfrancis.com
Taylor & Francis Verlag GmbH, Kaufingerstraße 24, 80331 München, Germany

www.ingramcontent.com/pod-product-compliance
Ingram Content Group UK Ltd.
Pitfield, Milton Keynes, MK11 3LW, UK
UKHW022017180926
475701UK00005B/888
9780367442071